Getting It

Getting It

A GUIDE TO HOT, HEALTHY HOOKUPS AND SHAME-FREE SEX

ALLISON MOON

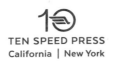

TEN SPEED PRESS
California | New York

"To cope with sexuality is difficult. Yes, but everything assigned to us is a challenge; nearly everything that matters is a challenge, and everything matters."

RAINER MARIA RILKE

"Be excellent to each other."

BILL S. PRESTON, ESQ.,
Bill & Ted's Excellent Adventure

CONTENTS

The Etiquette of Getting It 157

Heads, Hearts, and Other Parts 207

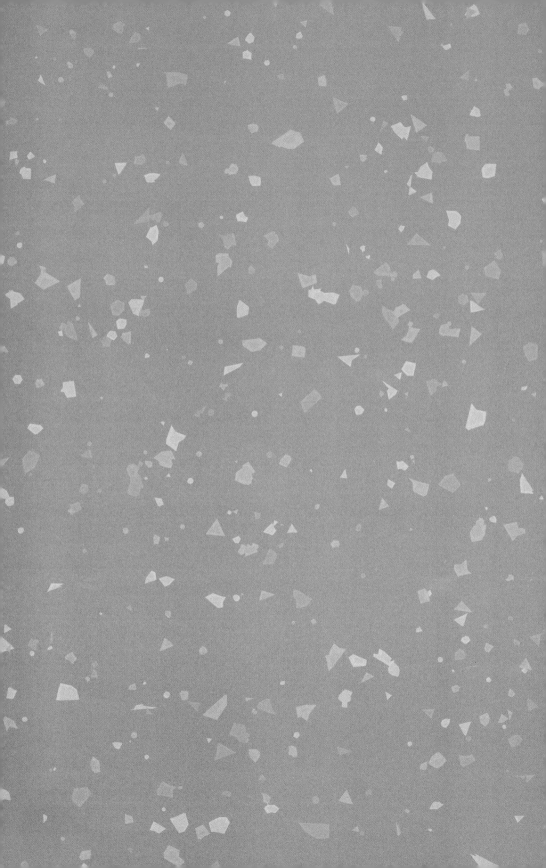

INTRODUCTION

When I was eighteen, I walked into my dorm room, agitated. I couldn't name the source of my frustration, but my (older, wiser) roommate saw the signs loud and clear. I was *horny*.

Of course I knew what horniness felt like, but this feeling was beyond the need to have an orgasm. It was *deeper*. I wanted to smell someone's hair, rub my face against their chest, and squeeze their muscles beneath my palms.

I wanted to *fuck*.

But I was still grappling with the lessons my parents taught me when they insisted sex was something to be shared only when you were in love (and preferably married; but let's be real, that wasn't happening any time soon). My high school sex ed taught me "Abstinence is the Best Choice!" My church taught me physical pleasure was suspicious and most likely sinful. Despite these warnings, I'd had sex with three people before I turned eighteen. Though, heeding my parents' advice, each was a committed relationship, and we were "in love" or some teenage approximation of it.

When I walked into my dorm, ready to rub myself against a tree like a grizzly bear, I was single and nursing a broken heart after Boyfriend #3 abruptly moved away.

I needed to get properly laid. Without a sweetheart, though, how was that supposed to happen? My roommate suggested I just go out and find someone to have sex with. I scoffed in prudish horror.

I'll never forget how she replied: "Allison, horniness is like hunger. It's a basic bodily function signifying a need."

Her friend agreed. "You're in college surrounded by other hot, single people. Go find someone to hook up with. Scratch that itch."

The permission those two women gave me changed my life. For the first time, I didn't see desire as love's by-product, but a perk of being a living, breathing human being. I could choose to work through the feelings in my body in another way, maybe through exercise or art. Or I could choose to go find someone cool to help me "scratch the itch." The choice was up to me.

I chose sex.

Since that night, I've had amazing sex with lots of wonderful people. Some of those people became lifelong friends. Some I never saw again. Each experience taught me something new about myself and people in general. Though I've gained lots of experience getting naked with people, I never stop feeling giddy, nervous, and thrilled when I get to do it with a new, wonderful person.

What Is Hooking Up?

Hey cutie,
Are you a 1972 Airstream with tow rig?
Are you my new Bluetooth-enabled 3-D printer?
Are you my new eco-friendly washer/dryer unit?
'Cause I wanna hook up with you . . .

Okay, so what is "hooking up" anyway?

The term has had many different meanings over the years. It's basically slang for "connect," which is why we *hook up* to the internet, *hook* our friends *up* with concert tickets, and *hook up* machinery to power sources.

Back in the old days, if you said you hooked up with someone, it often meant having full-on sex. In my wayward youth, it meant some sort of fooling around. Nowadays it can mean anything from a date to cuddling to sex. I believe the ambiguity of the term is its strength. Because all we're really trying to do is connect, sexually or otherwise.

In the rest of these pages, I'm not going to stress about the nuances of the term. Instead I'll share some advice on how to hook up honestly, happily, and drama-free.

Sometimes I'll use another complicated term: *casual sex*. What makes casual sex *casual*? What makes sex *sex*? It's a fraught subject, raising issues of morality, pleasure, risk, trauma, and choice. My job is not to convince you one way or another, but rather to give you good information to use to make up your own mind. I promise I won't shame you for your choices, and I hope you don't shame other people for theirs.

For the purposes of this book, here's what I want to aim for when I say *casual sex*. Casual sex is, ideally:

→ **Sex for sex's sake.** Casual sex ain't about making babies or doing relationship maintenance.

→ **Pleasure-focused.** Casual sex centers the pleasure of everyone involved.

→ **Collaborative.** Everyone involved is bringing something to the table. No one is a passive receptacle or disengaged bystander.

→ **In the moment.** Casual sex isn't about what comes next. It's about the present moment and what everyone decides to make of it.

→ **Equitable.** Everyone's desires, opinions, and needs weigh equally during a casual encounter.

→ **Community-aware.** Good casual sex respects the health, safety, and well-being of everyone involved, which in turns builds healthier communities.

→ **Exploratory.** Casual sex is an improvisational kind of sex, where we get to learn about ourselves, new people, and new concepts of play and pleasure.

Sound utopian? Sure. But it's an ideal worth aiming for.

With these values in mind, casual sex can be an antidote to our culture's hyper-regulated ideas of sex. Casual sex is sex that takes place outside the institutions of state- or church-sanctioned marriage. It's sex that seeks to undermine a transactional model of sex. It's sex that attempts to rewrite gender stereotypes. It's sex that revels equally in fancy hotels and dark back rooms, in wild orgies and hushed whispers. It's sex that declares its own intrinsic value, not as a commodity but an *experience*. When done well, casual sex stands up against hierarchies of power and their attempts to control our bodies and our access to pleasure.

In short: When you do it right, there is nothing casual about casual sex.

In a BDSM context, a good hookup can mean you feel *safe* feeling *unsafe*. You feel *respected* even as you are *disrespected*. You feel *appreciated* by being *humiliated or insulted*. BDSM and kink don't negate these tenets. In fact, they rely even more on their ever-presence. BDSM is a layer of context added on top of these basic criteria, not something removed from them.

In the following pages, you'll see my advice on how to scratch your itches in thoughtful and affirming ways. We're going to talk about consent, booze, STIs, love, orgasms, finding hotties to roll around with, and lots more.

My promise to you right now: I won't shame you for wanting sex, even if it doesn't come with a ring (or a second date!). I'll do my best to give you tips for making sure everyone has a good time.

So, let's take a ride through the wonderful world of hooking up!

Who Am I?

Oh hi, I'm Allison Moon. I've been teaching sex ed to adults for over a decade. I also write books, which I hope is somewhat obvious at this point.

My last book, *Girl Sex 101*, was all about how to please women, from the perspective of a woman who endeavors to do that very thing (that's me!). I wrote *this* book because I wanted to help everyone have better manners in bed, regardless of orientation or what they're packing in their panties.

See, I've been having sex with people for over twenty years. I've been in a blissfully nonmonogamous (and pretty slutty) partnership for thirteen of those.

I've done it with people across the gender spectrum. I've done it with people with varying abilities and limitations. I've done it one-on-one and in big ol' groups. I've done it with people I've known for five minutes, and I've done it with people I've been friends with for years. I've done it with people who didn't speak my language, and with people who never even asked my name.

Point being, I've clocked time with different kinds of folks, and I thought I might help you shorten your learning curve a bit in figuring out your own sex life.

I'm also kind of shy. I've got some body issues. And I've got an assorted mix of anxieties and challenges and strengths, like all humans do.

I'm white. I'm queer. I'm able-bodied and pretty "neurotypical" but not entirely. I'm gender-indifferent which gets read as cis, and I'm okay with that. I was born into a loving working-class family in the American Midwest (colonized Erie and Osage lands, to be specific). I grew up Catholic; now I'm an atheist. While I endeavor to represent complexity and investigate personal blind spots, I cannot escape my points of view, though I constantly work to expand them.

I wrote this book not because I'm some sex guru, or even particularly prolific, but because I've seen lots of really excellent sexy-time behavior, and some not-so-good behavior.

I've fucked up, too. I've hurt people's feelings. And I've been fucked over and had my feelings hurt. I think I have some good ideas about how to avoid this, and how to help set things right when situations go sideways.

All said, despite fuckups and anxieties and woes and regrets, I still have a great sex life filled with wonderful humans who are all busy having the sex lives of their dreams, too. So I think I have some good stuff to share.

Who Are You?

I don't know your gender, your age, your race, your religion, your orientation, your bodily configuration, or anything else about you. I expect there is no single trait that unifies everyone reading this book except for one: you give a shit.

You give a shit about yourself and about the people you sleep with. You give a shit about the world we share, and the unique challenges we all face trying to connect in it. You give a shit about the pleasure, health, and well-being of the people you meet (and hopefully even the people you'll never meet). That's it. I just need you to give a shit, or else this book is meaningless.

If you're an entrenched narcissist or a self-absorbed douchecanoe, you're not going to get much from this book. I'm not going to teach you how to trick people into having sex with you or manipulate them into vying for your affection.

Because here's the trick: There is no trick. If you don't give a shit about yourself or your partners, this advice won't work. It's really that simple, but that doesn't mean it's *easy*. In fact, giving a shit—all the time, in all the right ways—can be pretty hard. There's lots to calibrate for: feelings, values, contexts, personal histories, timing. In the next 200-odd pages, I'm going to help you learn how to track for those things. Some of it will be eye-rollingly obvious to you. You may have been eye-rollingly oblivious to some of it in the past. That's okay. A lot of this stuff we're still figuring out. We're just trying to get better at being excellent to each other as we go.

One more thing: This book is *not* a contract. You can read the whole thing and decide it's not for you, or you can pick and choose, based on what feels like a good fit. I implore you: **Take the advice that works for you and chuck the rest**. We're talking about *your* body, *your* heart, and *your* mind. So *you* are the expert. Some of this stuff may not resonate, some of it may piss you off, and some of it just won't apply to your life. Focus on what feels true to you and your unique tapestry of emotions and personal ethics.

My only request is that you read with an open mind and an open heart, with the goal that you want to deliver more joy and pleasure into the world, for yourself and others. Information is power, but when paired with self-love and empathy it becomes a superpower. Learn about yourself. Decide for yourself. Have fun.

— What Does It Mean to "Get It"? —

Sex is complicated. When we get naked with other people, we don't leave any of our baggage in the hall closet. We bring it with us into bed: our cultural context, our anxieties, our desires, and our traumas. Every bad breakup, every humiliation big and small, every moment of deep connection, every time we tried something new and it just didn't work out—it comes with us. Sometimes it's all very easy to ignore, but sometimes it can demand our attention, even when we're trying to focus on the fun bits.

"Getting it" means you understand that sex is complex and everyone has a different relationship with it. Approaching partners with sensitivity, curiosity, and compassion makes sex hotter, more connected, and more fun. It also makes *you* hotter, smarter, and more likely to attract a broad range of friends and sex partners.

A person who gets it:

→ Understands that each sexual encounter is unique, and different bodies need different things to feel good

→ Values the pleasure and physical, emotional, and mental health of everyone involved, not just themselves

→ Is patient with themselves and their sex partners

→ Does the necessary self-work to be safe for lovers to engage with

→ Takes responsibility for their own emotions, communication, or lapses of communication

→ Interrogates their personal biases about sex (including what is "too much" sex, what is "too little," what makes a good sex partner, what is good sex, and who deserves sex)

→ Understands why some people may have a hard time speaking up in and out of bed

→ Listens carefully to their partners before, during, and after sex—not just to words spoken, but to body language, silences, and energy

→ Accepts "no" with grace and respect

→ Respects their partners' freedom to engage, to change their minds, and to call things off

→ Works on understanding power dynamics, in and out of the bedroom

→ Respects other people regardless of attraction

→ Fights for sexual and reproductive justice for all

What I hope to do with this book isn't just help you get laid tonight, but teach you how to be a better sexual citizen. See, one of the biggest impediments to people not having casual sex is not feeling safe to do so. Safety is about more than being free from violence. It's about being free of slut-shaming, name-calling, neglected feelings, and poor treatment. When we get better at treating ourselves and our partners as worthy of respect and appreciation, we make it safer for everyone to fully explore their sexuality. And, surprise, surprise, this means more people get laid.

Creating a healthy hookup culture is in our hands. We can envision our ideal world and our ideal sexual self-expression, and we can take right steps to get there, together.

Getting Yourself

Before you get freaky with other people, it's good to know who the fuck *you* are. Part of being a responsible sex-positive person is knowing that no one is going to read your mind. No one is going to "just know" if you like something or not. It's your job to speak up and share the stuff your partners need to know. So before we dive into partnered shenanigans, let's spend some time getting this stuff on lock.

Who Do You Think You Are?

The first thing to figure out before pursuing a hookup is why you want to do it. There are plenty of great answers, and some not-so-great answers, but they're all valid as part of your journey. These might include:

- → The thrill of the hunt
- → A need for touch and closeness
- → To feel sexy and desirable
- → Adventure and stories to tell
- → To get over an ex
- → A desire for intimacy
- → A desire to *avoid* intimacy
- → Stress relief
- → Community building
- → Curiosity
- → Affirmation of sexual or gender identity
- → Pure lust
- → Escapism
- → Practice

- → Spiritual practice
- → Loneliness
- → To prove to yourself you can do it
- → To prove to someone else you can do it
- → To feel cool or accepted
- → To spite your conservative and/or religious upbringing
- → To make money
- → Revenge
- → You want someone who isn't available for a relationship beyond sex
- → To heal trauma or learn how to feel safe with sex
- → You just dig sex—you love variety and bodies and humans

Looking at the list above, circle the ones that sound like you, or write your own list on a piece of scrap paper. Try to be excruciatingly honest and really "feel into" your answers. You may find your responses illuminating. Some reasons on this list may seem more noble, joyful, or affirming than others. In fact, some of them are downright harmful to both yourself and your partner.

The important thing is to be honest with yourself about your reasons. Understanding your desires will help you be more intentional about your choices, getting you better results. For instance, if you want to prove to yourself you *can* have casual sex, but after trying it you don't find it gratifying, you can check that box and then let it go. If you're just horny and looking for a willing partner, be crystal clear with your prospects so they can choose to opt into a no-strings-attached romp.

If your reasons fall on the more harmful side of things, consider this your wake-up call to start treating yourself and your partners with more compassion and respect.

Overall, if you're finding casual sex unfulfilling, it may be because you haven't figured out exactly *why* you're doing it. You might be using casual sex where something such as an artistic outlet or nonsexual friendship could be more effective.

Among the many virtues of hooking up with different people is my personal favorite: VARIETY. But it's not just variety for variety's sake. Learning about different people helps you appreciate the amazing diversity of bodies and better understand yourself. You learn what pleasure *means* to people. Just because two folks might have the same equipment or gender identity, doesn't mean they enjoy the same things, like *at all.*

Just as travel gives you insight into different cultures, sex can introduce you to new worlds of touch and pleasure. I've been at it for more than two decades, and I'm still learning new things about how people like to have sex. For some folks, learning how to give one person pleasure is plenty, and anything more sounds exhausting. If that's you, great! Find that one person you want to give pleasure to, and forget the rest. If, however, you're keen to embark on a wide-ranging journey of sexual exploration, be prepared to have your mind blown (and possibly blow some minds yourself!) with the endless variety of bodies and pleasure.

Casual sex can also offer another more inward way of exploring variety. Everyone you're intimate with will see something different in you, awakening new parts of yourself. Others may remind you of things you might have forgotten about yourself. Sexual discovery doesn't end when you meet "the One" or hit a certain age. It can be a constant unfolding exploration.

Physical pleasure is a great reason to have sex, and sometimes it's the only reason. I applaud that. The world needs more genuine pleasure. It also needs more healing and companionship and expansion and creativity and love—all of which you can manifest in what some might call a "casual situation." There's no reason why you can't experience deep joy and giddy fun for one night with a person you'll never see again. Some of my favorite sexual experiences were with people I never talked to again. We had different paths, different goals in life, and different places to be.

Personally, I'm a big fan of having revelations in passing: "Hey, friend, thanks for teaching me something deep and heretofore unknown to me. I understand myself and my place in the world a little better having known you for the past hour. I sincerely hope you have a wonderful life."

I'm not kidding—it can really feel like that.

When done right, sex can make people feel a little less lonely, a little more appreciated and understood, and a little more worthy of love. So embrace the spectrum of what casual sex can be and the ways you can learn, grow, share, and connect with a partner and with yourself.

That's me. *What about you?*

I want you to think about your sex life and answer some questions.

You can write down the answers or you can just say them aloud. Either way, I encourage you to answer in concrete terms and project them outward. That is, don't just answer in your head and move on. A big part of good sex is being able to articulate desires, so why not practice right now?

Take a minute and reflect on your sex life until this point:

→   What have you liked most?

→   What have you not liked?

→   What do you want more of?

→   What do you want less of?

→   What has sex taught you about your body and your desires so far?

→   What would you improve upon?

Did you answer? Go on. Answer. I'll wait . . .

Good!

Now, this next part is vital. I want you to take a couple minutes. Relax. Imagine your **Ideal Sex Life**. It's okay if this feels weird or pervy or greedy. Just roll with it.

Is it you in the center of a monthly orgy? Starting a cam site with your bestie and getting paid to bone? Having a couple of sexy friends you see on the regular? Having one primary partner but enjoying a threesome every once in a while? Hiring a different sex worker each week to explore your fantasies? Having enough confidence to approach and flirt with new people? Being a free agent just hooking up when you wanna without shame?

Whatever it is, get the details down. Think about the people, frequency, locations, and energies behind it all. Once you've got it, answer these questions:

→ What kinds of *relationships* do you want with the people you sleep with? Friends with benefits? Anonymous and fleeting? Strictly professional? Something else?

→ What kind of *sex* do you want to have? Silly and playful? Kinky and nasty? Group or one-on-one?

→ What about this fantasy excites you?

→ What concerns or fears does this fantasy arouse?

→ What curiosities does this exercise pique? Does it bring up any things you'd like to try and/or learn in bed?

Keep in mind, sex is an individualized thing. Avoid language that assigns universal meaning to it. So, try to answer these questions with "I statements." For instance, rather than saying, "Casual sex is emotionally empty," try: "I'm afraid casual sex may make me feel emotionally empty." It's also a good idea to focus on what you can control. So rather than, "If I'm open to casual sex, so-and-so will like me more," consider, "If I'm open to casual sex, I'll have more dating options."

Remember, this can all change. You might think you want something and then have a change of heart once you experience it or contemplate it longer. That's okay. Just like we can periodically evaluate where we're at in terms of our career ambitions or any other aspects of our lives, it's a great idea to consider your sexual ambitions when designing your life.

THE CASUAL SEX BILL OF RIGHTS

The best way to draw the most positive aspects of casual sex into your life is by knowing and affirming your rights. The Casual Sex Bill of Rights can guide you through your casual sex journey. It will help you maintain boundaries and find partners who will rock your world.

1 The Right to Negotiate Your Terms

Any agreement you make, explicitly or implicitly, may be negotiated and renegotiated.

2 The Right to Your Pleasure

Pleasure moves through everyone differently. You have the right to get what you need to make it happen.

3 The Right to Not Be Slut-Shamed

If your sex partner slut-shames you, you have the right to call them on it and/or find a new sex partner.

4 The Right to Call It Off

At any time, for any reason, you are allowed to end the relationship/hookup/scene.

5 The Right to Have Feelings

It is normal and healthy to have feelings when you have sex. There is nothing wrong with having feelings. It means you are a Functioning Human Being™.

6 The Right to Have Fun

You're allowed to enjoy sex simply for the fun of it.

7 The Right to Your Reasons

There are *a lot* of reasons to have sex, only one of them being pleasure. As long as you aren't hurting anyone, and the sex is giving you what you need, then Godspeed!

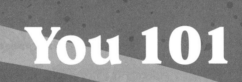

You 101

When you understand yourself, it's easier to write dating profiles, make small talk at parties, and describe what you're about and what you want. It also makes communicating in bed much smoother. This is especially true if there are quirks or nuances about things you like or don't like. This is *especially* true if you have any triggers that could derail the hotness.

So, sharpen your pencils, it's time for another exercise!

What are your pronouns? She? He? They? Something else?

What do you like your genitals to be called? Dick? Cock? Pussy? Vulva? Something else? If it changes, what is it dependent on? If there's a word that freaks you out or turns you off, let your partner know. This is especially important if using a certain word would misgender or otherwise hurt you.

What other words do you love or hate being called? You may be surprised how many women hate being called "lady." Are you one of them? What about "baby"? Sir? Femme? Stud? Some words may turn you on, but others may take the wind from your sexual sails. Sometimes it's contextual. (Only a few people get to call me Daddy. But those who do? SPLOOSH.) Sometimes you learn to like words you used to hate, or vice versa based on who's saying them or why.

What are your No Zones? If there's a body part you don't want touched, tell your partner up front. For instance, feet are a huge erogenous zone for some people and squicky to others. Know what you hate, and be ready to discuss it. Take care not to judge other people's likes. Don't squick their squee!

What's your STI status? What are your safer sex protocols? You should be able to share anything about your health that will directly affect you partner, including communicable sexually transmitted infections (STIs), and any rules for safer sex you have. For more on how to figure this out for yourself, see page 192.

What's your relationship status? Single? In an open relationship? Monogamous and cheating? These all have their own risks (both STI-wise and emotionally). Sharing your relationship status is part of informed consent and helps your partners navigate expectations.

What are your turn-ons/turn-offs? Does dirty talk make you feel silly? Will hair-pulling rev your engine? It's just as important to share turn-ons as it is No Zones. You don't have to share a complete list, but it's helpful to have a few of these in mind so you can help your partner know how to proceed.

Any communication preferences? If you have a preferred safe word, or there's something about you that could be considered alarming (like if you shift in energy in a specific or intense way when you're aroused), share it up front.

> When I'm in bed with a new person, I always tell them, "To me, 'Ow' means Ow." Which is to say, I like some pain, but if I say "Ow," I've reached my limit, so they need to dial it back. Anything until "Ow" is okay. This works in two ways: (1) they know they can get a little rough with me if they feel inspired and (2) they can trust me to speak up if I need to, which can help them relax.

Practice answering these questions out loud. The awkward, giggly answers are even more important to practice. If you can't say this stuff alone in your room, how can you expect to say it when you're getting naked with a cute person? *Practice.* Then bring these to your friends and practice with each other!

Keep in mind, your identity is not a recipe. Butch bottoms exist. So do straight guys who like sucking cock, lesbians who sleep with cis dudes, trans men who love their vaginas, kinky people who like tenderness, and on and on. Humans contain multitudes. Sharing your identity label doesn't actually say anything about how you like to fuck. Be clear.

If these questions were difficult for you to answer, you may need to do more self-investigation. Develop a curiosity about yourself, your sexuality, and your pleasure. Use that curiosity to open an inquiry into who you are and what you like. How?

→ **Read.** Check out the Recommended Reading on page 270 for suggestions. Follow interesting, sex-positive folks on social media.

→ **Meet people.** Expand your social circle. The more people you know, the easier it is to find dates. A diverse circle of friends also helps you learn more about yourself and the world, and that's just a good thing.

→ **Talk big.** My favorite part of small talk is when it leads to BIG TALK, like conversations about art, spirit, heritage, and human existence. Some folks are scared to indulge in such topics, but it's often where the juiciest bits of self-knowledge come from. Foster relationships with people you can get deep with, by practicing being conversationally and intellectually intimate with your friends. This, in turn, will help you be emotionally and sexually intimate with your partners.

Build Your Own Road Map

One of the hardest things for people to discuss during sex is what they actually want. A big part of this is shame and fear of ridicule/rejection. A less-appreciated but still-significant reason is many of us just aren't sure what we like in the first place. Between porn, mainstream entertainment, and cultural expectations, it can be hard to find an inner sense about what you specifically want. Figuring out what you like takes time, energy, and, most of all, *curiosity*.

Sexual pleasure has two main pillars: the Sensual and the Erotic. The **Sensual** is what *feels* good to your body. For some people this might mean the light touch of fingertips, for others it's the crack of a leather strap. Some folks love the blend of pleasure and pain. Others lean toward either edge. It's about what makes your nerve endings sing "More, yes, more!" The **Erotic** is what gets your *mind* going. It's the scenarios, the way someone looks, the power dynamics, or the idea of a sex act that gets you hot. These two pillars have significant overlap, and everyone has their own mosaic of what works for them. Exploring your own proclivities can help you suss out what you want in bed.

Masturbation can help you discover what you like sensually and, deeper than that, it's a good way to consider your entire relationship to sex. Next time you masturbate, give yourself twice the time you usually take. If your usual routine is jacking it for three minutes before you run out the door, try giving yourself a little more exploratory time before you bring it in for a landing. Try new moves on yourself. Emulate the touch you have liked from other lovers. If you don't masturbate already, there's no time like the present. Put this book down and start blazing a trail. There are few sensations a partner can generate for you that you can't do yourself with your hands or a well-chosen sex toy. So if you like partnered sex, you can certainly like masturbation.

The main practice with masturbatory recon is to **try new things**. Flick, twist, tug, and rub in a bunch of different ways. Explore more than just your genitals. Buy a new toy and take it for a spin. If you usually masturbate lying down, try it standing up. If you usually use your left hand, try your right. When you're exploring, stay present with your body. It's natural to want to lose yourself in the fantasy. That's awesome. But! Take the time to notice the sensations. Your nipple likes it when you flick it a certain way? Noted. The Magic Wand is way too buzzy for you? Into the giveaway pile it goes. This information is gold when it comes to sex. It gives you the chance to make your current and future lovers into sexual rock stars.

The main difference between simply jacking off and taking time to explore sensuality is the creativity and interest you invest. Maintenance orgasms are great. I jack off daily in the same way I stretch when I wake up. Exploratory masturbation is about connecting with my body and pleasure. It's more like doing yoga or meditating. Both maintenance orgasms and exploratory masturbation are good for you, so give yourself time and permission to practice both.

If masturbation helps you understand what you find sensual, **fantasy** can help you unlock your idea of the erotic. What do you think about to give yourself a sexy little jolt? When you find a fantasy that turns your crank, deconstruct it a bit. Let's say you have a naughty professor fantasy. You're a student who *really needs that A*, but Hot Professor thinks you just haven't done the work. You could earn that grade in other ways—wink, wink; nudge, nudge.

Okay, we're onto something. Now ask yourself, "What about this is hot to me?" It could be the power dynamic, or the fact that you once had a hot professor in real life who you still like thinking about. It could be the outfits, all plaid and tweed. It could be you're attracted to doing something forbidden and needing to be quiet so no one overhears your "office hours." There are a ton of ways to interpret this fantasy. Take time to examine these things for yourself and find out where your turn-on is.

This stuff is priceless when you're seeking out sex partners. If you realize your professor fantasy indicates you're attracted to intellectuals, for example, it may be a sign you should trade sports bars for book clubs to find the sexy-time match of your dreams. Deconstructing your fantasies is also a great skill for negotiation. For instance, if you want to play Hot Professor with a new sex partner, but that scenario just doesn't do it for them, you can propose alternate dynamics based on the underlying elements of the turn-on.

If you're feeling adventurous, here's a fun game to help build your road map: Look up porn that isn't what you normally go for, then try to find something hot about it. This allows you to expand your understanding of situations people find sexy, and possibly open up whole new realms of turn-ons.

It's okay if your disgust response kicks in here and there as you play this game. If that happens, you can click away. Or you can stick with it and tell yourself, "Some people find this hot. What about it could I relate to?" If this feels too edgy, look at written erotica or slashfic instead. While some erotica can be just as intense as porn, it's often easier to dip your toes in.

I once dated someone who was into humiliation. As a dyed-in-the-wool kind person, it's hard for me to get in the frame of mind of being verbally cruel to a person I like, even within the negotiated boundaries of a scene. How did I deal? I scooted on over to the internet and looked up erotic humiliation stories, particularly those told from the submissive's POV. The narrative aspect helped me to see the turn-on from their perspective. I understood the power dynamics, and how to wield them in a way that felt both safe and satisfying.

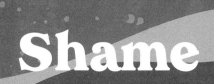

Shame

Sexual shame usually comes from a belief that you're abnormal for your desires, or if you were a better person you wouldn't want or do the things you do.

We can be shamed (by others or ourselves) for whom we're attracted to, what we fantasize about, and how we fuck. We can be shamed for having "too much" sex or "too little" sex. Rarely does the shaming correlate to our *actual* sexual habits, but rather the assumptions that people make about our sex lives and integrity, or the expectations we place on ourselves.

The first thing to know is you're not alone. We all, even the most libertine among us, have our hang-ups. Whether it's the fear of being unloved for our desires or believing we're not capable of enjoying what we have, lots of us deal with some form of sexual shame all the damn time. So give yourself, and everyone else, a break. We're all in this together. Even if you're one of the lucky few to have little internalized shame, understanding how it works can make you a better lover, friend, and partner. So let's dissect it, shall we?

Sexual shame is a cycle beginning with a dominant cultural message that's internalized by the people of that culture and used to police their peers. At its most effective, sexual shame only needs an occasional nudge by those in power to keep it circulating through a community. At its most extreme, sexual shame encourages people to join hate groups, enact freedom-restricting legislation, and commit violence against those who stimulate their feelings of self-loathing. Sexual shame prevents victims from reporting sexual crimes, talking frankly with friends and lovers about their desires, and acknowledging and healing their trauma. It is, to be perfectly frank, what keeps us from being fully self-actualized humans.

Be careful, though, not to conflate shame with guilt. Guilt is a common, rational, and generally healthy response to crossing a boundary or causing harm. Shame, on the other hand, is an internalized belief that you are deviant, broken, inferior, or unworthy. Put more succinctly: **Guilt is "I did a bad thing"; shame is "I *am* a bad thing."**

As much as shame can cause pain, it can also feel safe. If you can blame your feelings on Satan, a bad upbringing, or some genetic mistake, it helps explain things that are often just inexplicable. You can pray for salvation or commit to abstinence. You can say it's not your fault or all your fault. You can reframe your desires as pathology, a disease to be cured or ignored. The problem with these "solutions" is that shame is never truly silent and hidden. Shame manifests. It festers. It reaches into your life and demands to be noticed, often as bigotry, depression, or substance abuse.

Many people live in a constant state of shame management, but I think the better path is to work to eradicate shame from your life and your community. It's not easy, and for most, it's a lifelong effort. The result—living a fulfilling, self-actualized and fully expressed life—is worth every ounce of effort it requires.

Slut-Shaming

American culture is obsessed with purity. Which is ironic considering how *impure* our society actually is. (I don't mean sex. I mean the way we treat ourselves, other people, and the planet.) Purity obsession is directly correlated to sexual shame, and part of that obsession is how many sex partners you've had, aka your "number." People of all cultures, religions, and philosophies can become obsessed with their number and that of their partner.

Women are most often shamed for having a "high" number because our society is obsessed with female purity. Men, on the other hand, are more often shamed for having a "low" number because our society equates sexual conquests with success and validation.

Here's the big take-away: *Your number doesn't fucking matter*.

Your number affects literally *nothing* besides than your ego. Not your health, not your genitals, not your soul. Your number doesn't make you a better lover, person, date, or dance partner.

One of the most pernicious results of obsessing over the number is slut-shaming. **Slut-shaming** is the act of criticizing or devaluing a person based on their sexual reputation (either real or perceived). It's a technique for controlling people's sexuality using retrograde cultural norms. Rarely does it actually condemn any specific amount or act of sex. Instead, it's a catchall way of telling a person they're bad, immoral, or worthless. People in monogamous marriages get slut-shamed, celibate people get slut-shamed, abuse survivors get slut-shamed, and children get slut-shamed.

Slut-shaming can be explicit: "You're such a slut!"

And implicit: "You just met him!"

It can victim-blame: "Well, what were you expecting?"

It can be disguised as concern: "Aren't you afraid you're going to catch something?"

Or envy: "Wow, I wish I could bed-hop as much as you do."

It can apply to desires: "Why would you let someone do that to you?"

Or presentation: "Do you really want to wear that?"

It leads to problematic and incorrect assumptions: "You have no self-respect."

It creates standards for exclusion: "You're bringing shame on our family."

We live in a sex-negative culture. The messages we get are cruel, victim-blaming, and disproportionately focused on women, particularly those with other culturally marginalized identities (people who are trans, queer, fat, sex workers, disabled, of color, etc.). The more marginalized you are, the more violent and dehumanizing the slut-shaming can be. Women are supposed to be consumable, sexy objects, while at the same time preserving the illusion of being incorruptible, pure, and virginal. It is—literally—impossible to win.

The men who get slut-shamed are also often those with intersecting marginalized identities: disabled men, queer men, trans men, sex workers, and men of color. For example, one of the most pernicious and deadly effects of male slut-shaming is the villainization of Black male sexuality. America's racist history has created a paranoid fear of Black men as more sexually voracious than other men. This stereotype is directly responsible for countless lynchings throughout American history and leads to intense bi- and homophobia against and within Black male communities.

When we hew to a narrow definition of appropriate sexual desire and behavior, we remove opportunities for everyone to be authentically sexually expressive. Anything outside of what counts as "normal" sexual interest, including kink, attraction to non-normatively attractive partners, or emotional vulnerability can lead to slut-shaming.

Slut-shaming is easy to spot it when it comes from politicians, police, and parents. It's harder to recognize when it comes from friends. Odds are, though, you've been slut-shamed by someone in your community. Heck, if you're reading this book in public, you may be getting slut-shamed *right now!* (Cue scary music.)

The preachers and politicians know what they're doing when they slut-shame, but your friends might not. Even sex-positive, progressively minded people can find it easier to judge others for their sexual preferences than to accept them without bias.

In fact, *you* might be the one doing the shaming. Perhaps you read something in this book that made you wince. Maybe you thought, "How could anyone *like* that?" This, as innocuous as it may sound, is a form of slut-shaming. I've caught myself slut-shaming people—even my partners—wondering how someone can enjoy a certain porn or kink, or have sex with a certain number of people in one day. This stuff goes deep and is often invisible. It takes work to excise slut-shaming from your life, but it's worth looking deeper within yourself to consider why you may be acting from a place of sexual shame.

Now that you know how to recognize it, here's how to do your part to defeat slut-shaming:

→ **Don't accept slut-shaming from your community.** If your friends talk shit about people (even celebrities) because of the sex they like to have, call it out and shut it down.

→ **Don't punch down.** "It's just a joke" rarely is. Seriously, dead hooker jokes or "Is that a man in a dress?!" jokes aren't funny. Don't share them and don't humor people who tell them.

→ **Catch yourself.** If you judge someone—silently or publicly—for expressing their sexuality, notice the story you're telling in your head. Are you envious? Or are you repeating a shaming message you've been told? If you hear yourself saying "I could *never* do that!" or "People shouldn't . . ." or any "icky" responses to a friend's sharing, you may be slut-shaming.

→ **Eradicate shaming words from your vocabulary.** If you catch yourself calling someone (including yourself!) "loose," "desperate," "whore," "easy," or "slut," in a way that isn't reclaimed, quit it.

→ **Reframe.** We don't shame people for visiting too many countries, for seeing too many movies, or having too many friends. Why is it a problem to have a large number of sex partners? Having a large sexual history means you have a wealth of knowledge about other people's bodies and desires. Experience is a virtue.

→ **Broaden your horizons.** If you're skeeved out by a practice that people genuinely enjoy, it might behoove you to do some research. You may find a new appreciation for your friends and the wide world of sexuality.

Here's a fun fact: Having lots of sex usually makes you better at sex. If you have intentional, thoughtful sex, you get better at learning people's bodies and accommodating differences. This is one great benefit of sleeping with sluts! So instead of shaming them, you should be thanking them for clocking so many hours to perfect the art of sexy-times!

CUCK-SHAMING

Anyone, of any gender, can experience the inverse of slut-shaming, too. To be **cuck-shamed** is to be perceived as "unfuckable" due to a lower number or atypical sexual preferences. Those less interested in sex are often called things such as *frigid prudes* (in the case of women) or *beta cucks* (in the case of men). As with slut-shaming, cuck-shaming isn't based on reality, but what people perceive to be out of the ordinary.

Cuck-shaming is big in the pickup artist (PUA) community. The ethos behind PUA is all about making your number as big and impressive as possible to dazzle other men with its turgid, throbbing—wait, what was I talking about?

Right, PUAs are obsessed with quantity over quality. Having amazing sex with the same woman twice is less important to them than having mediocre sex with two different women. I hope it's self-evident why that's a bullshit and emotionally bankrupt philosophy. But cuck-shaming isn't only the domain of PUAs. In fact, sex-positive communities can be guilty of making people feel bad about their disinterest or lack of experience in sex, too. Be careful not to mock your peers or use sex positivity as an excuse to bully people into having sex they don't really want.

* * *

Whether it's slut-shaming or cuck-shaming, the end result is to punish people for expressing sexuality outside the rigid, narrow, and often arbitrary norm. Shamers have so much internalized shame that they need to externalize that self-loathing onto other people. Internalized shame can cause us to treat our partners poorly after sex, blaming them for our own feelings of self-hate.

When we internalize the shame doled out by our politicians, elders, corporations, and peers, we make it easier for them to control us. It can take a lifetime to liberate ourselves from shame. Some may instead succumb to it, subverting desires, quashing fantasies, or redirecting sexual energy down other vectors, some positive and some negative.

Our collective history is filled with ancestors who were denied their right to pleasure, joy, and a fundamental ecstatic practice. Many were even killed for pursuing it. More were persecuted or exiled. This wasn't the case for every culture, but most of us have a history of sexual trauma; if not in our personal lives, then inherited from our families. Intergenerational trauma is a real thing, with practical and painful repercussions.

How can you interrupt this legacy of shame?

Change your point of view. If you grew up in a highly religious and/or conservative environment, work to expand your horizons. If you have the ability to travel, do so. Even traveling to the nearest big city is often enough to help you realize how not-alone you are. If you can't travel, use the internet to find alternative communities. Read books about other people's sex lives. Listen to podcasts, like *Bawdy Storytelling* and *RISK!*, where people share true stories about sex. Try to love the diversity of humanity and find a space for yourself in the massive quilt of the human experience.

Interrogate the source and challenge its message. We don't emerge from the womb fearing our sexuality. In fact, infants (and even fetuses!) self-pleasure all the time. Who taught us to fear or hate sexual pleasure? What's their agenda? Who stands to benefit from you hating yourself and your community?

Deconstruct your context. If you're particularly inquisitive, you may find solace in deconstructing the reasons behind the shame you feel. If you are in a conservative Christian environment, for example, you may appreciate understanding the influence of the Church in imperialism, and how religion is used to uphold political power structures. If you come from a family that prizes female docility and compliance, it may help to examine why your culture historically hewed to that structure. None of us is immune to the ways race, class, and power influence how we have sex. I can't tell you how to deconstruct these structures for yourself, only to notice that they're there and be willing to interrogate the assumptions endemic within them.

Even if you didn't have a conservative upbringing, it's important to acknowledge that Western culture is pretty pleasure-phobic on the whole. We're taught to feel shame for indulging in purely rewarding activities. We feel "naughty" when eating chocolate cake, we think we're being "bad" when we call in sick to enjoy a beautiful day. To fight sexual shame, stop thinking like a productivity-prizing CEO and start thinking like a self-loving citizen of the earth.

Many people let shame dictate their choices without recognizing it. This is one reason why people with lots of shame often abuse drugs and alcohol. Substance abuse serves as a way for the subconscious to go after what it wants without letting shame derail the process. Practice interrupting self-destructive patterns or mindless choices by slowing down and taking time to question what you're doing.

Even the most liberated among us can run face-first into shame from time to time. What separates the pros from the amateurs is how much grace and love we give ourselves even when we get sucker-punched by our shame. Notice it, deconstruct it, and try to let it go. Learn to enjoy your body and its capacity for pleasure. Treat yourself as well as you'd treat a beloved friend. Be generous with the time and energy you give yourself. Explore hidden parts of your psyche. Love yourself *because of* not just *in spite of* all your nuances and desires.

It's okay to be a little embarrassed by sex. It's intimate! You make weird faces and sounds! It's kind of ridiculous in general! Nevertheless, practice gratitude and presence with your friends and lovers. Talk to people about their experiences. Be brave about sharing your own. You may find new, amazing friends and communities, and you may even create deeper friendships with people you already know and love.

If you know that sexual shame is interfering with your happiness, consider finding a professional to help you work it out. My strong recommendation is to find a sex-positive therapist. If you're kinky, queer, and/or nonmonogamous, make sure they have competency in those topics, too (see Therapy, page 247).

Remember: You're allowed to seek and have the sex you want. You don't have to stick to the cultural narrative you were born into. You are allowed to choose your partners, choose to be celibate, choose to be slutty, choose to be monogamous, and choose to have sex solo or in groups. You have the right to have consensual sex as often as you want, with whomever you want, regardless of what any preacher or politician says. True, you may have to leave behind your religion or your neighborhood to make that happen. That's your choice, too. Every day, all over the world, people choose their inner rightness and desires over what their community dictates. I won't pretend it's easy, but sometimes it's the easier choice when compared with living a life that isn't really yours.

Making Good Choices

When you open up to the idea of sleeping around, you'll realize quickly there are lots of choices to make. Swipe left or swipe right? Approach them or wait and see? Set up a date or text for a little while?

So let's talk about making good choices. (Note: I'm not calling these *healthy* choices, because I don't think the right choice is always the healthiest, and that's totally okay.)

Keep your intention in mind. *Why am I doing this? What am I looking for? What am I hoping to get?* This could be based on what you want from your life, or on the individual relationship between yourself and your partner.

Listen to your intuition. *What does my gut say? What is my inner voice telling me?* If you're always fighting against circumstance—if communication constantly goes sideways or you're always questioning your choices—it can mean something isn't in alignment with your intuition.

Honor yourself. *What's the advice I'd give to myself?* Many of us (sex educators included) are way better at doling out advice than we are at taking it. So practice offering yourself advice as though you were a beloved friend. If you saw your bestie making a terrible choice, how would you approach them? What would you say?

Draw from prior experience. *What have past experiences taught me about this choice?* In many parts of our lives, but perhaps particularly with sex, we develop patterns. We keep dating those jerks who remind us of our dad. We try again and again to get the prettiest girl to notice us just to prove something to ourselves. Consider your patterns in sex and dating. Is there one type you're always attracted to, even if it's irrational? Do you always end up in the same situation, or having the same fight? Do your friends respond to news of your dating life with a weary "Again?" If so, you may be playing out a subconscious pattern instead of making an informed choice.

Critical thinking. *How does this choice fit in with what I know about myself and what I want to experience?* Sometimes you just need to take a step back and evaluate your options with a critical, objective eye. Granted, it's not easy when the heart and/or genitals are involved, but it's a good idea to try. Take yourself out of the situation, detox from the hormonal cascade, and then assess what is the best choice. You don't need to be a shrink or PhD to be able to logically assess whether something is a good idea or not.

Focus on the feelings. *How do I feel about myself after we hang out/ I engage in this behavior?* Feelings are wily critters. They can trick you, lead you down strange paths, or hide truths. They can also reveal deep insights you might not want to believe. If you feel like garbage when you're with a certain person, if every time you do a certain thing you hate yourself afterward, if you're constantly second-guessing your choices, your feelings may be trying to tell you something your brain is trying to ignore.

Think big. *How does this choice fit in with my overall growth and happiness?* If you're aware you're working some stuff out, or want to explore a certain kind of experience, you can make choices that may seem odd to an outsider. A word of caution: Using other people for healing is tricky business. Sometimes your need to work stuff out can supersede your ability to treat the other person as a human being. It's okay to opt into relationships that are about your healing, but don't lose sight of the needs and desires of your partner in your search for enlightenment.

Own it. *How can I take responsibility for my choices?* Your job is to make choices you can feel good about. "Good" here doesn't mean morally superior or even, let's say, *constructive* choices. What it means is you make choices with a clear enough head to know when your choice is your own and when it's not. When it's not is when there's addiction, coercion, or nonconsent involved. In those instances, I recommend seeking help, in the form of therapists, lawyers, friends, or trusted community members. But you're allowed to make sexual choices that are edgy, risky, or scary. Get the risk-assessment formula (see page 188) ingrained in your head. Develop a working relationship with your self-esteem. Learn to trust your instincts. Honor your emotions. Listen to your intuition (instead of your shame).

Making good choices is an intensely personal experience. Take care not to use another person's sexual expression as a blueprint for your own relationship with sex. What may be one person's great idea is another person's anathema. The important part is to heed your own head and heart and make choices based on all the information and intelligence you have.

Intuition

The most foundational element to making good choices is learning to listen to your intuition. Intuition is the voice that says "This feels right" or "Something's off about this." Maybe you use another word for this: inner voice, Spidey sense, better angels, etc. Intuition isn't instinct, though. Instinct is a patterned response based in self-preservation or ego-maintenance. Instincts can serve a valuable role in getting you out of bad situations, but they can also lead you to make choices based on fear rather than growth. It's okay to listen to both, but pay more attention to your intuition, as it is often quieter and slower than your instinct's quick reaction.

Intuition often feels like clarity and certainty, and it can lead you toward things that resonate with or excite you. It's a feeling, deep in your core, about what you want in your life. It's an inner sense of rightness that no religion, guru, parent, or ideology can touch. The better you get at listening to your intuition, the more decisively you can opt in or out of things, and you'll likely feel more confident in your choices.

Developing your intuition requires practice. This is one realm where folks with a spiritual and/or meditative practice may have a leg up. Practice listening to your intuition with these exercises:

→ Recall a time when you knew exactly what you wanted and took decisive action. Maybe it was to take a job, move, break up with someone, or come out as something. Recall the feeling of making the decision. Did you feel it in your body? Was there a clear voice in your mind?

→ Think of something about yourself you just know to be true. I don't mean about the world, I mean about *you*. Feel into it. What does that knowing feel like in your body? How does your mind react to the assertion? It's okay if your brain starts concocting logical stories or throwing up contradictions to go with the assertion. Try to sense the difference between the deep knowing part and the logical loop-de-loops.

→ Meditation is good for you. When you're able to quiet your mind and control the flow of thoughts, it is easier to hear the tiniest voices in the deepest parts of your brain. Once you've gotten good, you'll find you can quiet your mind even when not in a meditative state, like when you need to make an important decision or when you feel overwhelmed.

Intuition feels *right*. Our logical brain often makes us second-guess ourselves. Our intuition, on the other hand, often feels like serenity and ease. When you make a decision, do you feel freaked out or calm? Search for the choice that feels true and creates an ease in your mind, and you'll likely be on the right track. If, for instance, you're trying to decide if a person is worth pursuing, ask yourself, "Do I like myself more or less when I'm with them? Do I feel better about myself or worse? Do I feel sexy or unsexy? Smart or stupid? Lovable or unlovable?" True, if you grew up in a toxic household, you may have some wires crossed when it comes to what makes you feel loved. Adult relationships (particularly casual ones) are great opportunities for you to practice feeling balanced and desirable, even when you're excited or nervous. Try listening to your inner sense of rightness, and you may find yourself moving toward a more compassionate relationship with yourself.

WHEN YOUR RADAR IS BORKED

Some of us have good intuition when it comes to sexy-time. We tend to choose good partners and have generally positive results. Meanwhile, some of us have no idea if we can trust our gut. We choose duds, have bad experiences, and are left wondering what the fuck were we thinking?! The most common reasons for a "borked" radar are a shitty upbringing or a traumatic past. This doesn't mean you're screwed, just that you might need to spend some extra time thinking through your choices.

Validate yourself. You'll get nowhere by telling yourself you're full of shit. A cycle of self-loathing just means you become your own worst enemy and fight against your inner voice. Practice giving credence to your thoughts and feelings rather than fighting or minimizing them.

Feel your feels. Our society places a weird amount of value on white-knuckling through tough situations. Denying our emotions is just flat-out unhealthy. Suppressed feelings find their way out eventually, and the longer you suppress them, the more likely the outburst will be harmful or destructive. We need to give ourselves permission to feel. That doesn't mean we have to act on every emotion, but we have to allow ourselves, even in baby steps, to sit with our feelings and listen to what they're telling us.

Interrogate your instincts. If you find yourself inexplicably drawn to someone, give yourself a moment to consider why. It may be they're just fucking hot and you're smitten. It may also be you're playing out an unconscious and potentially unhealthy pattern.

Pump the brakes. Adrenaline is great fuel for making rash choices. If you're feeling a shit-ton of pressure to Decide Right Now, take a break, take some breaths, and let your blood chemistry calm down first.

I had a BIG crush recently. It made me feel loopy and anxious, but in a fun, gaga kind of way. I'm usually a pretty even-keeled and reasonable person. So when I started second-guessing myself and feeling insecure, my friends and lovers were suspicious. It turned out this guy mirrored seriously toxic behaviors from a past abusive relationship. He simultaneously evoked all the giddiness *and* all the insecurities of my seventeen-year-old self. Once I noticed the pattern, I knew I needed to start resolving my old wounds instead of committing to new ones.

WHEN YOU FUCK IT UP ANYWAY

Sorry to break it to you but you're probably going to fuck up anyway. You'll ignore your intuition, dive head first into the bed of a bad fit, or play out some shitty old pattern you've spent years trying to escape. So what then? How do you manage when you make the *wrong* choice despite your intuition?

Self-correct as soon as possible. Remember: You're allowed to change your mind. Sure, course-correcting can be weird, awkward, or just plain difficult, but it may be well worth it. You'll thank yourself later.

Forgive yourself. One of the worst parts of making the wrong decision is feeling like an idiot. To the degree you can, forgive yourself. You made a choice based on the information you had at the time. Maybe that information was skewed by a traumatic past or inebriation or peer pressure. Chalk it up to a learning experience, figure out what lesson to derive from it, and move on.

Internalize the lesson. Once you've identified the wrong choice and forgiven yourself, try to open an inquiry into why you made that choice. Too often we get stuck beating ourselves up so we don't take time to learn from our mistakes, which all but guarantees we'll make the same mistake again. So take your time and think through future scenarios where you can make a better choice.

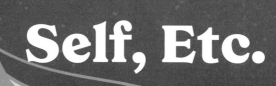

Self, Etc.

A good way to assess your choices is with a whole bunch of "self-" terms you may recognize: self-esteem, self-confidence, self-concept, self-awareness, self-care, self-love, and self-actualization.

We all have a different relationship with these metrics. For example, it's possible to be self-aware but lack self-esteem, or to have high self-confidence but be uninterested in self-actualization. Awareness of each term is important because they affect the choices you make, including choices about sex.

→ **Self-esteem:** The positive regard you have for yourself. When you think about yourself, are you a fan? Do you *like* the person you perceive yourself to be? If you have high self-esteem, you're likely to choose partners who think highly of you as well. If you have low self-esteem, you may choose partners who "prove you right" by treating you poorly.

→ **Self-confidence:** Your belief in your capabilities and aptitude. Do you believe you're a capable person? Are you able to learn, adapt, and accomplish things? Do you feel fit to navigate the challenges of day-to-day life? If you have strong self-confidence, you believe you make good choices and can handle different situations. You're generally okay with spontaneity and trying new things. If you have weak self-confidence, you don't take risks or try new things. You don't trust yourself to make good choices.

→ **Self-concept:** The way you evaluate and perceive yourself. Are you able to describe yourself in clear terms? Can you reflect on yourself and feel secure in the accuracy of your vision? If you have a strong self-concept, you know who you are. You can try things on for size in your mind and have a sense of how you'll react in real life. If you have a weak self-concept, you often feel like a stranger to yourself and choose partners who are a bad fit.

→ **Self-awareness:** Your capability for introspection assessment of how you feel, think, and react Do you understand how your mind works? Can you rely on your instincts and intuition? Are you aware of your challenges, fears, and anxieties? Does the way you see yourself tend to line up with how your loved ones see you? If you have high self-awareness, you trust your intuition to be correct, and you know how you'll react in different kinds of situations. If you have weak self-awareness, you second-guess your choices, accept other people's incorrect assessments of you, and let people bully or coerce you because "they know better."

→ **Self-care:** How well you tend to your needs. Do you know what your body, mind, and heart need to feel good? Do you know how to restore your reserves when you're depleted? If you're good at self-care, you have an arsenal of things you can do to tend to yourself. You know when you need to take a break or lavish some love on yourself. You know when social/sexual time will be nourishing versus depleting. If you're not good at self-care, you burn out, put everyone before yourself (even to your detriment), and can grow to resent yourself and others.

→ **Self-love:** How much you love yourself and in what ways. Do you make healing and caring choices for yourself? Everyone makes the occasional self-destructive choice, but on average, do your choices make your quality of life better rather than worse? If you have a lot of self-love, you make healthy and nourishing choices. You respect your body, mind, and spirit and expect the people in your life to respect you as well. If you have little self-love, you may make harmful, destructive choices, shut out other people, or invite harmful people in.

→ **Self-actualization:** The desire to reach your fullest potential. Do you have goals? Do you consider what you'd like to accomplish in life? Do you have a clear value system you can look to in times of discomfort or confusion? If you have high self-actualization, you're less likely to make choices (such as having high-risk sex) that could interfere with your goals, and you're more likely to choose sexual experiences that are in alignment with the person you want to become. If you have low self-actualization, you don't have much ambition and don't consider the future when making decisions. You may be prone to choosing harmful or self-destructive options.

* * *

You probably resonated with some of the previous descriptors, either on the positive or negative side. Some things you may have been working on your whole life, whereas others you never thought twice about. I don't expect I'll get you from shitty to awesome, but even small changes in your decision-making can have significant, positive effects on your life. Here are some ways to start.

Upgrade your friends. The influence of our friends *matters*. In high school I was a theater nerd, which meant I spent Friday nights belting out show tunes instead of raiding liquor cabinets. Nowadays, I'm less about the show tunes, but I still have great friends who think I'm awesome and smart and funny. And you know what? *I believe them*. When I'm having a shitty week, my friends lift me up. When I need to process relationship drama or get a gut check, I have them for that, too. Find friends who do the same for you and strive to be that person for them. Ask yourself, if I make a choice to improve my life, how will my friends react? Will they support me? Or give me shit? If I need some TLC, who shows up? Who can't be bothered?

Note your strengths. Good at keeping plants alive? Make a damn good scone? Got booty for *daaaays*? Doesn't matter what it is, just recognize it. Abusive parents usually cut their kids down and make sure they don't get "too big for their britches." If you grew up in a household like that, you may need to practice crowing about your talents. Start now! Write down three things you're good at. They can be anything, as long as you're proud of them. Then tell yourself, "Hey, me. I'm awesome at _____, _____, and _____. Good job. I'm proud of me."

BONUS: If you're internet dating, you just got a head start on your profile!

Honor your body. Go on a stroll, do stretches, turn on some music and rock out. Respect your body, even if it's got some issues. It's what you've got to work with, so give it some love. Move, breathe, and feel good.

Masturbate. Self-pleasure is a form of self-love. Even if you don't orgasm, self-pleasuring is good exercise. Practice breathing and feeling all those delightful endorphins flow into your bloodstream. Relax and let your body receive some joy.

Help others. Another tried-and-true method for improving your sense of self-worth is by serving others. This can be in the form of volunteer work or just calling a friend to see how they're doing. Sharing love increases love.

Replace self-critique with positive affirmation. This can be tricky, especially if you grew up in a household where you were constantly criticized. Negative messaging can hold on tight, but you can always get better. Practice replacing self-critique with a neutral or positive self-assessment. For instance, instead of "I'm such an idiot!" go with something like, "I've never done this before and I'm learning," or "This is challenging, but I can handle it."

Act with good intent, and assume good intent from others. Some of us were raised to be suspicious of kindness or generosity, so we don't trust people who treat us well. Many folks assume the worst of others, thinking it protects them. The fact is, the opposite is true. Most people aren't monsters. When you assume the worst in people, you isolate yourself, and your suspicions can become self-fulfilling prophecy. Your thought of "They don't want to hang out with me" becomes true, because you've pushed that person away. If you assume good intent, you allow yourself the opportunity to actually get to know people. If they turn out to be jerks, then you can get them out of your life, but at least you know for sure! Same goes for you: act and speak from a place of compassion and love. Life is hard, man. Everyone is dealing with shit in their lives, most of it invisible to outsiders. If you can be that person who offers others a little bit of respect, dignity, and compassion, you'll start to offer that same stuff to yourself, too.

We all have bad days, and some are worse than others. Some of us struggle with depression or chronic pain. Some of us can barely get out of bed each day. My advice is not intended to diminish the real hurdles many of us have to deal with on a regular basis. The key is "progress, not perfection." Patterns can be hard to interrupt and self-improvement takes work. Give yourself patience and permission to be clumsy. If you need help, find a therapist, doctor, or group that can offer it. I truly believe these things are the golden ticket to great sex, great love, and great lives. You just have to give yourself permission to practice.

Sexual Empowerment

Sexual empowerment is the ability to make choices for yourself around your sexual attitudes and behaviors. "Empowerment" has become somewhat of a marketing buzzword, but it basically means you feel capable, responsible, and sovereign over your sexuality. Empowerment comprises a few things:

Authority. You are the ultimate authority when it comes to decisions about your body and heart.

Skills/Knowledge. You understand your body. You have a variety of ways to give and receive pleasure. You are open to new things and upgrading your skills.

Resources. You have access to information and support around your sex life. This can be community, health care, and fact-based education.

Responsibility. You can take responsibility for the choices you make, both when victorious and less-so.

To improve your sexual empowerment, start by taking stock of all the ways you feel empowered and disempowered. Look at the following list and check the ones where you feel empowered and circle where you need improvement.

→ I control my reproduction.

→ I have access to health care.

→ I have friends I can talk frankly with about sex.

→ No one else tells me when I have to have sex.

→ I can give myself sexual pleasure without having to rely on a partner.

→ I know at least three resources for accurate sexual information.

→ I understand STIs and how they are transmitted.

→ I can use the STI protocols I want to with my partner(s).

→ I understand basic sexual anatomy.

→ My sexual partners honor my boundaries.

→ I don't need to use alcohol or drugs to enjoy sex.

→ I am my desired level of "out" regarding my sexual and gender identities.

→ I can speak up when something isn't working for me.

→ I know what kind of sex I want and how to ask for it.

→ I have places I can go where I can be myself.

→ I have people who help me feel sexually self-expressed.

→ I have healthy/supportive nonsexual relationships.

→ I know how to apologize to sex partners I may have hurt in the past.

→ I am proud of my sex life.

There are no right or wrong answers here. Your responses will simply help you get a sense of where you could shore up your sexual empowerment.

For most of us, sexual empowerment is a lifelong process. There's no gold star when we check off all the boxes. Like with any self-improvement journey, it's about progress, not perfection. So see where you can take small steps to improve your sexual empowerment and get started today.

Loneliness

Loneliness is a response to isolation, sometimes physical isolation but more often social and mental isolation. We can feel lonely in crowds, surrounded by friends, or even when we're the center of attention. Loneliness can be *existential* ("we're born alone and we die alone") or it can be *conditional*, like when we're missing just one important person, when we feel ostracized from a group, or when we feel alienated from ourselves.

In general, our brains delineate boundaries, creating a separation between self and everyone/everything else as a means to make sense of the world. When we're in love or feeling intimate, that clear delineation between self and other dissolves a little and allows us to feel seen, validated, and maybe a little less lonely. This means that when we're isolated from intimacy, the chasm between self and other can feel vast and brutal.

Folks who self-medicate to curb feelings of loneliness are often looking for this temporary dissolution of boundaries, using their drug of choice to feel less alone. A more sustainable method of dealing with loneliness is to deconstruct it into beliefs and interrogate each one. For example, your loneliness may have you believing you aren't special or you're too weird to be loved or too mediocre to be interesting. Interrogating these underpinning beliefs may help you identify needs, which you can then turn into requests that you can start attempting to source from the world.

Another technique? Have a life. I know that's some basic-bitch advice, but it's really fucking important. When you are at your loneliest, when you feel most isolated and unlovable, there has to be *something* to get you to put on clean underpants and get out there. Maybe wobbly, maybe anxious, maybe unprepared for the thousand little paper cuts the world doles out on the daily—go anyway. Social isolation is horrible for mental and physical health. Even a brief nice interaction with a person on the bus has more of a positive impact on mental health than social media does. And yes, this is true regardless of your gender and whether or not you consider yourself an introvert.

Also, try to be of service. Volunteer work or even just helping a friend can help you realize your validity in a world that feels indifferent to your existence. Remember we all need people, and you can be there for someone who needs you.

Finally, own up to it. Dating and sex are the most obvious things we do to feel connected to one another. If you invite a sexy friend over to help stave off loneliness, there's no shame in being honest. You may find they accepted the invitation for the same reason.

LUST AND LONELINESS

Like hunger, desire is a signal, a little ping in our brain that says, "Your body needs something." There's little to fear here. We get hungry, we eat, and all is well. What can feel scarier is when our hunger becomes starvation, when we wonder if we'll ever eat again, or when we contemplate the lengths we would go to to feed our needs.

Most of us are familiar with the feeling of wanting sex but not being able to get it, for whatever reason. Even worse is when hunger for sexual touch tips into starvation. It can make us feel desperate or angry. It can make us feel out of control, or subject to the whims of whomever we desire.

This is, in a word, dangerous. When lust can't be satisfied, we may blame those we desire for not "feeding" us. We think we deserve sex and others are being cruel or callous for denying it to us.

I don't know how to fix this on a global scale, but we need to start by acknowledging the pain. It's okay to yearn for something you don't have. But, remember, it's not anyone's fault. No one owes you their body, ever.

Find other ways to feel good. This could mean taking up hobbies or a spiritual practice, or just moving your body in affirming ways. People are attractive when they enjoy their own company. So start there.

Feeling good requires platonic touch, too. Particularly in American culture, and particularly among men, there's little cultural permission to touch one another. It causes a real phenomenon known as "skin hunger." People need touch. We just do. So find ways to fill up your touch tanks. Get a massage, go to a Cuddle Party, take a dance class, play some full-contact sports.

To get your needs met, consider hiring professionals. This could mean a talk therapist, a massage therapist, a professional cuddler, or a sex worker. There is no shame in paying people to provide a service other people get for free. When I dated a hairstylist, I got free haircuts. After we broke up, I was back to doling out $60 for a trim. *C'est la vie*. The bonus is: Money creates boundaries and offers opportunities for exploration. So if you just need some loving touch, why *not* hire someone for that?

Sexual Resiliency

When we enter the world of sex and dating, we open ourselves up to a world of hurt: rejection, heartbreak, microaggressions, boundary violations, and difficult conversations. Yet most of us still walk headlong toward the source of pain, knowing that the hurt is worth it. Welcome to intimacy, folks.

One of the best things we can do as individuals searching for love, connection, or intimacy is to cultivate resilience. Psychological resilience is a person's ability to cope with difficulties. **Sexual resilience** is a term I use to describe that same quality within the realm of sexual relationships. Because sex comes with so much baggage, even if we're resilient as heck in our "normal" lives, it can be harder to be sexually resilient.

Cultivate flexibility. Rigid things break more easily. Flexibility can help you avoid getting sucked into the quagmire of rigid expectations. Try to go with the flow when possible. Remember there's almost always a third option (and a fourth and a fifth). Don't get stuck on either/or thinking. Cultivate intimacy or sexual fulfillment in other ways than the one you most want. Aim to create win-wins for everyone involved.

Educate yourself. It can be hard to make good choices when you don't know what your choices are. If you don't know what other ways there are to pleasure a vulva other than penis-in-vagina sex; if you don't know where to buy non-latex condoms; if you don't know how to talk to someone who uses gender neutral pronouns—FIGURE IT OUT. Develop curiosity and then feed that curiosity. It'll serve you for a lifetime.

Develop self-awareness. Did something hit you weird? Maybe a comment or a sort of touch made you feel off? Note it and figure out what about it threw you. It's possible the other person stumbled into a pain point you didn't know you had, or knocked into a boundary you never articulated.

Foster your ability to move on. Some of us deal with bad news or experiences by distracting ourselves: shoot some hoops, get drunk with friends, or get out of town for a few days. Others tend to mull and dwell. Both strategies have their strengths, but try to strike a balance. If you're a mover-on-er, make sure you give yourself adequate time to feel your emotions first. If you're a dweller, practice getting yourself up and out, into a world of moving the fuck on.

Have a menu of self-care options. Diversify your options.

Surround yourself with resilient people. It's hard to be around dwellers, mopers, and eternal victims. Rather than get stuck in the quagmire, cultivate friendships with people who can handle mistakes and setbacks with some grit and humor. It's okay to get thrown, but it's helpful to have support systems, too. If you need help upgrading your resiliency, spend time with friends who can support you on that quest.

Flirting and Finding

So you're ready to dip your toes into the hot, horny waters of hooking up. Great! The hard truth is, most hooking up involves other people, which means you need to *meet* other people. Have my fellow introverts curled into the fetal position yet? Yeah, for many of us, it's the *least* awesome part of hooking up. Flirting with a hottie you're pining for can make cunnilingus with a pillow queen feel like a freakin' cakewalk. So, let's dive face-first into the face-melting agony of flirting.

Hottie, Hook Thyself

One of the biggest myths about sex is that the only people getting it are the conventionally hot ones (or, barring looks, the rich ones). This isn't true.

The fact is, people of all shapes and sizes, of all ages and backgrounds, get laid. While mainstream culture would like to pretend there's a narrow definition of "attractive" that only the white, slim, and young inhabit, attractiveness is actually remarkably diverse and only partially influenced by social conventions.

The key isn't to attract people. It's to *be attractive*. I know that sounds odd, but bear with me. Read on to learn how to get your feet (and other parts) wet.

How to Be Attractive

If you're worried about not finding cuties to fool around with, the best place to start is with yourself. Pick up a hobby, develop a skill, learn a new language (or two). All these things have a dual benefit of making you a better person while also making you attractive. Sure, for some folks that might mean getting to the gym more, but it's only really effective if you love the results! If you hate exercise, spending two hours a day in a gym will make you miserable, which will make you miserable to be around. If you love you some kettlebells, however, and you like people who are attracted to developed lat muscles, then by all means, that's a viable direction.

You know that saying, "Life is what happens to us when we're busy making other plans?" Well, *hotties* are what happen to us when we're busy doing awesome things. For some that might mean traveling the world with Doctors Without Borders. For others it could mean having an interesting job, cultivating fun hobbies, or having a group of friends who enjoy doing things together. Having a life will bring more hotties into your sphere, but even if you don't connect with most of the people you encounter (and let's be honest, most of us don't), you *still have a life*.

The key is to find a thing that lights you up—something you *want* to get good at and brings more joy into your life. For instance, I knew a girl in college who learned American Sign Language so she could volunteer at a local Deaf services organization. The added benefit was she could communicate with some superbly hot people whose own hookup options were limited by a language barrier. Reach out, learn some stuff, meet some cuties.

Next, flag that shit! Flagging is a nonverbal communication system developed by gay men to advertise what they're into and what they're looking for. You may have heard of it as the "hanky code" wherein certain handkerchief colors denote different sexual proclivities. Simply think of flagging as advertising what you're about. All humans, regardless of orientation or gender, send signals about who we are. Our hairstyles, our clothes, the various ways we adorn our bodies—we're sending messages. If you think you're "true neutral" in the way you dress, I'm here to tell you, that's a choice, too. So make sure the choices you're making are sending the right message. Style yourself to advertise who you are. When you amplify and broadcast your own intrinsic qualities, you attract people who like those qualities about you. Then, miracle of miracles, you have surrounded yourself with people who enjoy the same things you like about yourself. Congratulations, you've created a self-love feedback loop that'll serve you for a lifetime.

There's a reason why musicians, actors, and athletes have a reputation for getting laid. Sure, they're talented, but the real reason is they perform their talents in front of literal crowds. They're advertising themselves being awesome *for a job.*

I'm not suggesting everyone has to start performing at open mics to get laid (please, God, no), but the takeaway is: Go out and do stuff *with and around other people.* This may mean setting up a local World of Warcraft guild where you go out to dinner once a month. Or start a book club, or teach coding at your local after-school program, or whatever. Enjoy your interests, but don't brick yourself up in a tower. If you want to touch people, you have to be touchable.

I know this is obnoxious advice because it's such a cliché, but your mom was right: Be yourself. Why? Because you're more likely to meet people who are into people like you by being, well, you. If you pretend to be into swing dancing because the girls are cute, but you really prefer speed metal, stop hanging out in the swing clubs and get thee to a metal club! Sure, you may end up sifting through a sea of duds, but it's better than dating someone whose hobby annoys the crap out of you.

Some people take to casual social situations easily, but many more people have some social anxiety. I sure do. There are lots of social cues to keep track of, and if you're awkward, into some freaky-ass shit, or just super-duper shy, being yourself can feel scarier than not. In this case, consider geeking out on social skills. Learn to make eye contact (which I know can be hard), track body language, and carry on polite conversation. Treat human socialization like any other subject you'd want to learn. This isn't to be manipulative or shady, but to be able to converse with people without feeling like a total tool. Develop skills to help ease yourself into feeling more comfortable meeting other people.

A super cute chick once told me she was nervous to talk to me, which is why she decided to break the seal and do it anyway. She had no opening line, no rehearsed follow-up, just, "I think you're sexy and you make me nervous but I wanted to say hello!" I wasn't sure how I felt at first, but I dug her endearing bravery. We got to talking, and yep, we totally hooked up and it was awesome. Good job, brave cutie!

Cultivate curiosity. Genuine interest in others is sexy. Ask good questions, and truly listen to the answers. Studies consistently show that the best and quickest way to connect with people is to ask them questions about themselves. Sure, some people may get nervous talking about themselves, but it doesn't mean they don't like being asked. Remember to pay attention to the rules of the environment. For instance, it's generally great to ask "How do you know the host?" and less so "Are you into bondage?" (unless of course, you're in a kinky space).

When it comes to curiosity and interest, people tend to either be snorkelers or scuba divers. That is, some folks like to stay on the surface and see lots of stuff. Others like to go deep. Both qualities are great, but when it comes to meeting people, snorkeling is a good way to go. While you may enjoy going deep into kung fu cinema, for instance, it may limit your conversation opportunities to people who share that specific interest. Consider picking up some knowledge on kung fu–adjacent topics, like different kinds of martial arts, action-filmmaking techniques, or East Asian historical movements. Expand your interests widely. This offers more opportunities to find connection and familiarity among people who may not share your specific area of geekery.

Some of us are born with the gift of gab. Others have a hard time with this kind of relating. Luckily, conversation is a skill you can learn, and even more luckily, conversation doesn't have to look one way. You may have to chat with someone for a while before you find mutually interesting conversation styles or topics. So ask questions and see what you can learn about one another.

Conversations are collaborative, just like sex. If a person dominates a conversation, asking few questions or offering little opportunity for the other person to speak, it can send a signal that they may bring those qualities into the bedroom. Explore conversation like you hopefully explore sexuality: with curiosity, generosity, and appreciation. You don't have to pretend you're competing for Miss Congeniality, but it's helpful to be a person other people want to be around. That usually means minimizing complaining and navel-gazing, fostering an interest in other people, and finding joy in all sorts of places.

Social anxiety, introversion, and good old-fashioned shyness can combine to emotionally hogtie us, so we never ever make a move. This can create a middle-school-dance scenario where everyone is waiting to be asked to dance. It takes courage to be the one to walk across the gymnasium and invite that cutie to boogie. Regardless of your gender, though, you're going to have to suck it up and be the one who approaches every once in a while. Just as fortune favors the bold, hotties favor the brave.

Flirting Fundamentals

Flirting is just getting to know someone, and being playful at the same time. Both sex and flirting are forms of play, so when you flirt with someone, you're learning if your styles of playfulness are compatible. Imagine flirting as a playground. Some kids are quiet and contemplative. Other kids are rambunctious and rowdy, running like wild. Some want to be the boss, and some want to be bossed around. No one is wrong, just different. As a grown-up, you're pretty much doing the same thing. You're simply looking for the adult version of someone you can play with.

The Art of the Approach

If you're shy, trust me, I understand. There's a reason why I write books instead of, I don't know, *meeting* people. I still get tongue-tied and too nervous to make a smooth approach. I can feel too loud or too quiet or too big or too invisible. I'm antsy and awkward and I still do okay, so I promise you can, too. Here are some simple ways to start.

Be sincere. Compliment them on something you genuinely appreciate. Like their style? Their hair? Their smile? Their taste in coffee beverages? Just say so. Odds are the object of your affection will be polite back, especially if you're offering a sincere compliment. If they're a jerk, whatever; they've probably cured you of your crush.

Be friendly. You're looking for someone to have fun with, not a hapless victim of your villainous scheme. Most people don't take too kindly to aloof, rude, or cruel people. So be warm, kind, and human.

Be flexible. Being attached to outcomes sets everyone up for disappointment. I've met some excellent friends through flirting. Some of them I was hoping to hook up with but didn't. Some of them I was hoping to hook up with and totally did. If you're not attached to outcomes, success can look like having a nice conversation, making a bunch of new friends, or just breaking through your anxiety and asking a cute person to dance.

Be choosy. We've all had the experience of lowering our standards when we didn't get what we wanted. Jobs, housing, a position on the sports team, whatever. Generally speaking, settling can be a perfectly fine tactic. However, hooking up is one of the few places that I encourage you to stick to your guns. Don't settle for your crush's friend, when you really wanted the crush.

The exception to this rule: If you suspect you have unrealistic expectations about yourself or the people you want to hook up with, it may be a good idea for you to examine your standards and find places to chill out a bit. Pining after nothing but supermodels won't usually get you what you want. Instead, start looking at people who look back at you. That's when things get interesting.

Be specific. Sometimes when we crush, we don't think beyond the goal of getting them to crush on us back. It's a good idea to have a step two in mind for what happens after they say, "You're cute, too." If you want to schedule a date for some other time (a particularly good idea if either of you are inebriated at the moment), or meet in the library for a make-out session, or just eat pizza and cuddle, being specific can garner great results. The fear of the unknown is what shuts a lot of us down. So articulate exactly what you'd like to do with someone, where, and when, and you may be pleasantly surprised.

BREAKING THE SEAL

Lines are for the bank, yo. There's a reason why all those cheesy pickup lines are used like jokes. They *are* jokes! Any pun, generic transparent flattery, or inauthentic posturing might get you a laugh or a groan, but what next?

Instead of behaving like an amateur actor cold-reading a script, and once the line is said, standing there like a fool, think more like an *improv* actor. The first rule of improv is "Yes, and . . .," which means you go with what the other person gives you, and you add to it. That's why improv is new each time. It's just a conversation, but to converse well, you have to *listen*. So give the other person an opportunity to respond by asking a question. It can be a silly question or an insightful one, something you're genuinely curious about or just something that's fun to ponder. Whatever it is, just be sure it offers room to respond. If there's only one right answer, and the object of your attention got it wrong, that's a dick move on your part. Instead, think about what's situationally appropriate and can lead to a bigger conversation. Disposition and personality matter *way* more than cleverness on a dime. If someone feels good being near you, it won't matter if you gave a witty retort to a slow pitch or stumbled over the punch line of a silly joke.

Overall? Just freakin' say something! Hanging back to run scenarios like some sort of X-Men-level clairvoyant won't do you any good. You have to connect. It needn't be brilliant, clever, or even cogent. You just have to break the seal. Getting shot down is an opportunity for closure. Instead of the big weeping wound of "What could have been?!" you'll get the "Eh, nothing will be. Moving on. . . ."

Crushes

Oh my god, they're so cute! Their smile just kills you, you want to bury your face in their neck, you want to smother them with kisses, and, and, and. . . .

You're amped up on adrenaline, oxytocin, and cortisol. You feel heat, energy, a little nervous tickle inside. You want to touch them, to smell them, to learn all about them. This is called *attraction*.

Attraction can be purely physical (something about their pheromones just gets you HIIIIIGH), physical with an added intellectual and emotional excitement (pheromones plus "What's your favorite movie and why?"), or it can be heavy on the emotions and intellect with just a dash of physical attraction. No matter how you cut it, you have a crush.

Crushing is healthy. You can have crushes while you're single, in a monogamous relationship, or playing the field. Crushes don't have to hurt anyone, and they aren't cheating. Nevertheless, it's common to get flustered when you're talking to a crush. That's just a sign you care. High stakes can create high anxiety. There's nothing wrong with feeling high stakes, especially when you're feeling big feelings. But remember to breathe and take your time. It'll help you listen and speak better, and take the edge off of performance anxiety. Some of us feel the need for speed when we're engaged in conversation. We want to be quippy and ready with a snappy reply. We want to keep the energy up and not allow for any lulls. I certainly understand the urge. I'm a hyper-verbal person, and when I get nervous I tend to motormouth. One thing I've learned is to give myself a chance to think. If I'm asked a question, it's okay to ponder for a moment to find the right words. It's also fine to stall. I've learned to say, "Let me think about that for a moment," or "I want to answer your question, but I'm having a hard time finding the words." If they're truly interested in you, they won't mind a momentary lull to gaze upon you adoringly.

Practice letting go of overanalysis. Humans are meaning-making machines. We *love* to try to make every small gesture into a big moment. While it's generally great to pay attention to details, it can be a problem when you assign meaning to those details. There's a difference between "He touched his mouth when he said that," and "He touched his mouth when he said that! Is he lying? Does he want to kiss me? Is he lying about wanting to kiss me?!?!?"

Notice the things you notice, but interrupt the script that takes you to "IT MUST MEAN THIS." In my experience, rarely are you right, especially when you're looking for evidence that you're not compelling company.

If you're getting caught in a spiral about whether or not they're actually enjoying the conversation, ask for reassurance. Something like, "I'm enjoying chatting with you, but am I keeping you from circulating?" Don't assume someone's always looking for an out, especially if it feels like things are going well. Avoid self-negging. It's another scientifically validated fact that folks really don't like hanging out with self-deprecating complainers. It's great to have feelings and be honest about yourself, but be careful not to let it tip into bitching about everything. If you're dealing with heavy stuff, it's okay to mention it, but be mindful of what's more appropriate for a therapist than a date.

When you feel anxiety, it's often because the part of your brain that feels fear has convinced you that you're in danger, even if it's just emotional danger. Use your logical brain to override your fight/flight response. Acknowledge you may be acting a little unreasonable. At worst, you'll get rejected by a person you like. It won't kill you. It'll hurt, you'll heal, and you'll move on.

Don't fib. Some folks lie or exaggerate when they get nervous. But lying is a deal breaker for lots of people. So if you make the silly mistake of saying, "Yes, I loved that movie" when you haven't seen it, fess up. It doesn't have to be some giant confession, just something like, "When I said I loved *Rashomon*, to be honest, I couldn't get through the first fifteen minutes. I just wanted you to think I was sophisticated." If that admission is enough of a deal breaker for the other person to bail, you did yourself a favor. In my experience, though, that kind of confession is rarely received with anything but a sweet laugh and a sincere "thank you" for being honest.

Finally, diversify. Don't put all your sex eggs (ew) in one basket. Keep your options open and keep flirting and meeting new people, even if you find one person you're super excited about.

CHEMISTRY LESSONS

The defining aspect of a crush is it's a one-way street. It's something you feel for another person, whether or not that person reciprocates, which they often won't. Unrequited crushes can be delightfully painful, or just plain painful, but they still help exercise your lust muscles. When a person *does* reciprocate your crush (lucky you), we enter into the land of chemistry.

Chemistry is when two or more people have a mutual attraction. It's a conversation, a dance, a shared energy. It's when they make you blush and you make them blush, too—or giggle, or flirt, or scoot a little bit closer. That said, chemistry doesn't have to mean anything. You can have chemistry with people who end up becoming your BFFs, basketball buddies, bandmates, or best friend's partner. You can have chemistry with people you never plan on dating or sleeping with. Or you can explore dating, sex, friends with benefits, or romance. It's all gravy, as long as everyone is on the same page.

If you're nervous about rejection, a good remedy is to stop pursuing attraction alone and instead seek out the two-way street of chemistry. There's nothing wrong with getting rejected (other than the fact that it hurts), but prioritizing chemistry can help improve your odds.

PRO TIP

Chemistry does *not* negate verbal consent. You still need to ask and get permission before you touch or escalate any sort of chemistry into the sensual or sexual realm. Chemistry is simply an indication—a temperature gauge, if you will—as to whether you wanna try to get that car on the road.

Awkwardness

"Okay, Allison," you might be thinking, "this is all well and good for socially apt people. But I'm awkward as hell. What about me?!" Which . . . fair.

For people with social anxiety or those who have a hard time reading social cues, flirting may seem more stressful than a solo mission to Mars.

The truth is, before you can be the super-stud you were meant to be, sometimes you might have to be a little dorky. Start by giving yourself permission to be like a baby deer, all wobbly and off-balance. With practice, you'll find your footing. Then, try the following.

Don't be afraid to lead with basic questions. Things like, "Hi, can I talk to you?" or "I don't know anyone here. Would you like to hang out?" are perfectly fine ways to break the ice.

Pay attention to verbal cues. Do they ask you questions about yourself? Do they answer your questions with openness? Do they give you compliments? ("You're funny!" "That's a great point." "You're the coolest person I've met here.") These are all good signs. Meanwhile, terse or noncommittal answers to open questions are usually a sign that the person isn't interested.

Learn to track body language. It can be hard to know what people are trying to communicate without using words. Pay attention to nonverbal signs of connection such as casual touch (a soft touch on your arm or scooting closer), eye contact (when talking and especially if paired with a smile), open laughter (there's a difference between a nervous laugh and a comfortable one), and body posture (the rigidity or relaxedness of their shoulders and stance).

Compliments are okay. Stick with nonsexual things beyond immutable physical appearance, such as the way someone speaks or answers a question. Compliments on personal physical choices are usually fine to break the ice: hairstyles, clothing, tattoos or piercings, etc. Things people can't control, like their body shape, skin color, or hair texture, often aren't a great starting place.

Be clear about yourself. It's okay to tell someone you have a hard time making eye contact or you're easily distracted in busy environments. Many people appreciate that kind of forthrightness. If they don't, it's probably a sign you two might not get along anyway.

If you're unsure, ask. People often use coded language when they're uncomfortable. Odds are you've heard a girl tell a guy "You're sweet" as a means of turning him down. If you're not sure if the person you're talking to is brushing you off in the same way, politely ask.

Adjust your expectations. A lot of us have unrealistic expectations of how often people connect. Sure, you may have a buddy who's always getting numbers, but that's much rarer than the rest of us who are thrilled if we meet one person we're attracted to every six months. Go into social environments with the goal to just have a nice time, and you'll likely to be less disappointed if you don't leave with a date.

Literalism can make people uncomfortable. Humans have developed innumerable ways to code communication to make things less literal. These codes can soften harsh language, foster politeness, and generally smooth uncomfortable social situations. This code can be hard to decipher, though. Ask for clarity when necessary.

The good news is, as people become more comfortable talking about neurodiversity, the spectrum, and personality variance in general, it's becoming easier to find matches—not always and not as fast as many of us would like, but it's happening. As usual, I recommend leading with the "scary" stuff first, and you'll likely have better luck finding someone who can hang with you, awkwardness and all.

What Is Creepy?

The word "creepy" is often used to describe people (usually guys) who approach people (usually women) in an off-putting or vaguely threatening manner. The stigma of the term has made many folks terrified of being called creepy. What is creepy, really? And how can you avoid being That Guy?

Creepy is being attached to an outcome. If you approach someone with the goal of sex and then find things are not going in that direction, you may try to steer things back to sex. This is creepy. If you get cranky when things go in a different direction and then start to resent the object of your affection because they aren't behaving the way you want them to, this is creepy. Being attached to an outcome means you want ultimate control of someone else's experience. You want to move them around like a video game character instead of giving them free choice to opt in or out.

Instead, do as our Buddhist friends do and practice nonattachment. Learn to be okay with another person's preferences and proclivities, even if they don't stack up to your hopes. Let people have their autonomy and choice, even if that choice is not to hang out with you.

Creepy is attaching your emotional well-being to a specific result. Deciding "I need to leave with three numbers or else I'm a miserable loser!" is a recipe for, well, misery. When we place the health of our ego in other people's hands, we create a needy, hungry vibe that can be extremely off-putting.

Instead, cultivate self-love independent of external validation. Yeah, easier said than done, but it's worth the work. When you don't need to get fucked to feel fuckable, get a date to feel datable, or get flirted with to feel flirt-with-able, you'll have a much healthier way of pursuing sex. A fun side effect is that not needing external validation is often precisely what gets it for you!

Placing your emotional needs in an external locus of control is almost always a recipe for heartache. The only thing you can truly control is yourself. So instead of thinking "I need three numbers to make this night worthwhile," consider a reframe such as "I want to approach one person I think is cute, no matter how nervous I get." That way, you're finding ways to validate yourself.

Creepy is not taking no for an answer. Here in America, we have a weird attachment to tenacity. I blame Hollywood. Romantic comedies constantly reward creepy behavior. Whether it's stalking, inappropriate declarations of love, or wearing someone down until their no turns into a yes—those things are creepy.

Instead, let no mean no. If you're gracious and kind when hearing no, sometimes people will change their minds, but only if you've heard and honored them to begin with.

Creepy is purposefully *or* accidentally ignoring another person's discomfort. Seriously, you can be creepy without even knowing it, and that sucks.

Instead, learn to pay attention to nonverbal cues. Is the person meeting your eye contact? Are they leaning closer or engaging you in conversation? Are they asking you questions and eager to hear the answer? Or, are they answering your questions with clipped, monosyllabic answers? Are they looking around like they're trying to find an escape? Are they answering your requests with "I dunno" or "I mean, I guess" or other noncommittal replies? Try giving people a gentle out and see if they take it. You may get all the information you need about whether someone is eager to spend time with you or not.

Creepy is believing there's some sort of secret code to get people to put out, and if you follow the formula to the letter, everyone will quiver before you.

Instead, acknowledge that humans aren't sexbots. There's no Konami code for getting someone naked. Some people will be into you. Some won't. That's life. Everyone goes through it. You're better off enjoying people's company, learning about them, sharing about yourself, and letting sexual affinity develop from there.

Creepy is hiding your intentions, with "Do you need a ride?" or "Want to come up for a nightcap?" If your intention is to get laid, using subterfuge to get what you want is creepy.

Instead, discuss it. If you suspect the person you're grooving on is sweet for you, too, ask them on a date, or say you'd really like to make out. If you don't know if they're attracted to you, find out first. Say something like, "I think you're cute. Would you like to hang out one-on-one sometime?" If they don't reciprocate, back off.

Creepy is needing to lower someone's status to feel good about yourself. "Negging" isn't sexy or flirtatious; it's preying on someone's insecurities to force them to try to win your approval. It basically makes you everyone's crappy, disapproving stepdad. I don't know many people who find that dynamic alluring.

Instead, be kind. This doesn't mean cheap flattery. Just be sincere and treat people with respect. You catch more flies with honey, and more honeys with honey.

Creepy is seeing what someone will let you "get away" with.

Instead, stop seeing sex as transactional, and start seeing it as collaborative. Pay attention to what you want to cocreate with someone as opposed to what someone will let you do to them.

Creepy is thinking that if you were hotter you'd get away with bad behavior.

Instead, realize that even if you look like Captain America or Wonder Woman, you can still be creepy. Using good looks to be a creeper is just shitty. Being friendly and kind will get you much further than chiseled features ever will.

Discomfort versus Offense

Among conscious, sensitive people, there's a concern on how to even approach a person you're attracted to. Often they say they "don't want to offend" someone. There's a distinction, however, between offending someone and making someone uncomfortable. It's normal to feel uncomfortable sometimes. Couch cushions can be uncomfortable. The dentist can be uncomfortable. Most of us are a little uncomfortable saying no. It's just hard to reject people. There's nothing inherently wrong with feeling uncomfortable, nor gently and respectfully putting someone in a situation where they have to say yes or no.

> "Can I skip in front of you? My plane's about to leave."

> "Can I borrow your cell phone? I have to make a call and mine's dead."

What separates discomfort from offense is how you listen to the answer.

Discomfort slips into offense when a "no" is ignored, when a power differential is exploited, or where silence is assumed to be assent.

If, for instance, I'm at a bar alone and want to stay that way, and a man offers to buy me a drink, I now am in the position of either rejecting him or not rejecting him and dealing with something I didn't want. So, I'm uncomfortable. He may be feeling uncomfortable, too, because he just hit on someone and is waiting for a response. Here we both are, together in our discomfort.

What happens next can tip it either way.

If I say no, and he says "Okay, thanks!" and goes away, the discomfort is generally mitigated. He might feel a little disappointed and I might feel a little flustered, but no harm is truly done.

If, however, he doesn't even bother asking if I want a drink before he orders one for me, now things are moving in a bad direction. He didn't wait for my opinion, he didn't care whether I'd say yes or no. He just did the thing he wanted to do without my consent. Now, I'm offended. Because he's established he doesn't actually care about my opinion.

Recognize the difference?

If he asked and I responded with silence and then he just went ahead and ordered, that's also removing my consent. Because in all things, sex and otherwise, **silence is not consent**. If I'm fumbling for my words or just taken off guard, I may need a moment to come up with a cogent answer. The best thing my hypothetical suitor can do in this situation is wait or ask a different question, which may be easier for me to answer, such as "Do you want company or would you prefer to stay in your book?"

True, culture dictates what's appropriate, too. In some places, it's considered gentlemanly to buy the drink first before asking. In this case, it's still key to listen to how the object of your interest responds. If they say "No, thanks," graciously take your extra drink elsewhere.

Here's how to make an offer without adding extra pressure:

→   Use your words.

→   Offer invitations; don't back people into corners.

→   Wait for a clear opt-in before engaging.

→   Don't touch people without their permission.

→   Don't equate silence with assent. Treat silence or a maybe as a no. It'll save you all a headache.

→   Don't try to negotiate. If you get a no from someone, don't try to find the exception. Just accept it and move on.

→   Lead with humanity. Objectifying people right out of the gate usually doesn't engender a feeling of safety. Start with something neutral so you can both figure out if you like each other first.

→ Don't take it personally. Even a brush-off may not be about you. Maybe that hottie had to deal with four other more aggressive dudes before you showed up. Take the brush-off, and chalk it up to their loss.

Advanced Flirting

Okay, now that we've got the basic moves down, I want to kick it up a notch and give you some tools for social awareness. Social awareness is a complex and nebulous concept that requires you to track multiple dynamics at once. So beyond "Does this person like me and do I like them back?" we're taking into account your context, power dynamic, and histories. The better you get at noticing the granularity of intersecting contexts, the easier it is to connect with people and help them feel safe with you. Deciding when it's appropriate to hit on someone is one of the hardest parts about modern flirting, and the fear of creating an awkward moment means many of us hedge.

First, note your context. Where are you? Work? The park? The gym? There are some places that are officially off-limits for flirtation. Other places don't have official limits, but are culturally inappropriate. Is it likely that everyone is safe? Does everyone have somewhat equal footing? For instance, a job interview ain't the place to hit on someone, bud. Save it for the dog park. Consider how the context interacts with your culture, too. I can't tell you what's appropriate for your specific subculture, but it's important to understand the rules you're playing by. For instance, hitting on someone at the gym is A-OK for most American gay men. But straight people? Nerp. Most women *hate* getting hit on at the gym. In some cultures, it's considered fair game to holler at someone from the sidewalk. In many other environments, that's offensive and creepy. Some social gatherings are designed with specific anti-flirtation rules in mind, while others are created with the sole intention of encouraging people to meet and flirt. Pay attention to the cultural space you're in and act accordingly.

Note the power dynamic. Some places, like school, don't prohibit flirting wholesale, but they do prohibit it between people of varying powers (for instance, teachers and students). But power isn't always as clear-cut. When you have a crush on someone, you often feel like they have power over you, no matter what your Privilege-O-Meter says. Even if you're a straight, white, rich guy, you might feel like that super-cute barista at your local coffee shop has power over you. It's okay to feel that way, but it's less okay to act as though your crush mitigates all the various differentials at play. When in doubt, if you're the one with more structural power in the situation, *don't pursue it*, particularly if that power differential means you have material control over their lives. This may indeed mean an attraction passes without ever coming to fruition. My opinion, in a word? *Good*. It's better to put the onus of pursuit on the person with less structural power in the situation or wait for that power dynamic to shift (e.g., they transfer to a different department, say, or you pay for the meal and get up to leave), rather than put anyone in a situation where they might put their job or safety on the line just by saying "No thanks."

The challenge with this advice is it places the pressure to make the approach on people who have historically been taught *not* to do so. In certain situations, it can actually be unsafe for a person of color, a trans femme person, or a gay man, for instance, to hit on someone with more structural power or an unclear sexual orientation. If you don't hold structural power over someone, *pay extra attention to the context of the relationship*, gauge everyone's comfort (especially your own), and proceed with care. Let them know you're interested or open, but won't get shitty if they don't feel the same way. Power isn't just one clear thing, and everyone will have their own tapestry of privileges and marginalization. You don't have to have complete mastery over social dynamics to be a responsible flirt. It's a good idea, however, to practice clocking differentials and adjusting accordingly.

As a sex educator, I often get booked to teach mini-classes before sex parties. It's kind of like the dance lesson before the salsa club opens for the evening. It's common for some attendees to get a little hot for teacher. There's a built-in power differential: I'm getting paid to speak as an expert, and they're paying to be there as a participant. My rule is I never hit on participants, but I'm open to them hitting on me.

At one such party, a woman approached me, disclosing she'd never been with a woman before and she wanted me to be her first. She was also Black, femme, and in her early twenties—a whole bouquet of power differentials. I told her I was open to playing, but we'd need to have a long talk first. She spoke with such control and certainty that I felt confident in her ability to assert her needs, so I agreed. We had a lovely time and she was a great communicator. Afterward, she asked for my help approaching another group of women, and I sent her on her merry way.

Preferences
and Taste

Dating can feel alienating. We might fear we'll never find someone who turns us on in the right way, likes the same kinds of things, and just "gets" us. The remedy sounds antithetical, but I promise it helps: *Get more specific*. I know, you think I'm full of shit. When it already feels like there's a one-in-a-million chance for you, how can being *more* specific help? Well, it's a signal-to-noise situation. Your specificity will allow your signal to cut through the noise of everyone else.

Be clear *what* you're looking for. If you want activity buddies, a quick romp, or someone to try that new restaurant with, be up-front about it. This also goes for specific kinds of sex you're looking for. If you're a straight guy who *loooves* getting pegged (hey, boy, hey), odds are good you'll find more compatible ladies if you state your interests up front. You may be surprised who answers the call. (The bonus is this can preemptively weed out slut-shamers who aren't down for the kind of play you're seeking.)

Be clear *who* you're looking for. Having preferences is important. If you just say, "Eh, whatever," you're going to get a whole lot of whatevers. Don't be afraid to ask for the kind of people you want. Specify gender if it matters to you, or be clear if it doesn't!

Be clear about who *you* are. This is your chance to weed out people who can't hang with someone as rad as you. If you have physical issues that make certain kinds of sex harder, if you have kids, if you have a job that means you're only in town every other month, share that stuff. It might mean getting fewer matches, but the ones you do get will be higher quality and more likely to be down with (and *go down on*) you.

Be up front about your *intentions*. If you just want to fool around and/ or go on dates, say so. If you're looking for free drinks, own up to it. If you like to string back-to-back hookups together, be real about it. There's nothing wrong with having sex with three different people in one night, so long as you're honest about it. Hell, some folks may get off on the idea of you hopping along to another bed (or inviting them all over at once!). Find the people who get off on the same stuff you do, and life becomes a whole lot more fun.

Stick to your guns. Don't compromise on big stuff because you're lonely. Sure, you may end up going on more dates, but if you're spending time with people who don't make you feel good, you may end up just as lonely.

If your only criterion for potential mates is a pulse, you may find yourself overwhelmed by terrible prospects. You're not doing anyone any favors when you cast too wide a net. Because, odds are, you *do* have preferences, you're just scared to choose, or you don't want to believe you're a judgmental person. Preferences save everyone heartache. If you *hate* that your sweetie isn't a vegan, and they hate that you hate that about them, no one's happy. If you avoided speaking up at the beginning of the relationship because you weren't honest with yourself about how important veganism is to you—guess what? *You're* the jerk in the scenario. Have your preferences, and be willing to stick with them, and you'll date people who thrill you instead of make you grind your teeth in an herbivoracious rage.

A word of warning: You get to choose your standards. You don't get to dictate other people's, particularly in casual arrangements where you're not merging households or making life decisions together. You can make requests, but you don't get to tell them how to live their life. If their personal choices upset you, consider whether your relationship is worth them not meeting that standard. It may be that you'd both be better off calling it quits rather than suffering through each other's disapproval and frustration.

That said, know that your preferences are not immune to critique. In fact, your preferences may indeed perpetuate cruelty, oppression, and harm. They may even be *products* of cruelty and oppression.

In cases such as these, saying "It's just a preference" doesn't give you any moral high ground. This is especially true if you espouse one set of morals (like body acceptance or anti-racism) to your friends, but practice another in the bedroom.

This goes for genitals, too. You can prefer people who are packing one set of goods, but remember, genitals do not equal gender. If you like people with vulvas, remember that most cis women, most trans men, and many trans women have vulvas. So what are you actually looking for?

Be willing to deconstruct your preferences and you may find that what you thought was a deal breaker wasn't such a big deal at all. Take care to not let stereotypes rule your sex life and discount potentially wonderful partners based on your unconscious biases. If you think high school dropouts can't talk philosophy or people with disabilities make bad dance partners, you've got lots more living to do, and lots more opportunities for connection than you think.

Chemistry is an odd duck. You often find it in places you're not at all suspecting. Give yourself the chance to find chemistry with people who may not look like what you were expecting. You deserve intimacy, you deserve pleasure, and you deserve to be seen for the great human you are. So does everyone else. Be open to finding sexiness outside of your normal paradigm.

— Win-Wins to Deal Breakers —

On a piece of paper, make four columns and label them: Win-Wins, Wiggle Room, Three Strikes, and Deal Breakers. You're going to go through each list and write things that apply in each column.

Win-Wins are exactly what they sound like. If a partner has them, everyone is happy. This could look like shared interests, shared values, compatible kinks, etc.

Wiggle Room are things that don't thrill you but aren't worth ending a potential relationship over. These can include bad habits or things you'd prefer were or weren't present but aren't deal breakers. Think about stuff your prior partners have done that didn't drive you wild but were fine.

Three Strikes are things that are close to deal breakers but you'll give them some slack to sort it out. Like if they smoke but they're quitting, or they aren't quite with it on a subject that's important to you but they're demonstrating growth.

Deal Breakers are "shut it down" moments. If a partner has/does them, you're out.

Here are some attributes to get you going. Try placing each one in a column. (If an item doesn't matter one way or another to you, just leave it off.)

→ Atheist	→ Sexually inexperienced
→ Bondage top	→ Weed smoker
→ Cat person	→ Polyamorous
→ Has kids	→ Religious
→ Closeted	→ Genderqueer

Sometimes we don't know something belongs on our list until we've had firsthand experience with it. For instance, I might think dating a smoker is fine, but after a couple dates, I discover it's actually quite off-putting. I might put that on my Three Strikes or Deal Breakers list. Similarly, you might think you could never date someone who's religious, but after connecting with a devotee or two, you may realize it's not actually that big of a deal after all. If there are

Deal Breakers or Three Strikes things that occur to you as odd once you write them down, that may be a good spot to interrogate a bit. You may find you were using a stereotype instead of relating to people as people.

Don't be afraid to be shallow, though! If someone being short or white or a parent or whatever is a deal breaker, be honest about it. If you're afraid of someone reading this list, put it in a password-protected document on your computer. The key is to be brutally honest. You never have to share this with anyone.

Hopes, Expectations, and Boundaries

Some people work hard to live their lives without expectations. There's a Zen quality to this—to lessen suffering by limiting the opportunities for disappointment. It's a noble ambition, but it's also rather unrealistic in interpersonal relationships.

If you get stuck in expectations, practice letting go a little bit. Every time you notice yourself getting thrown by someone else's choices (or lack thereof), investigate whether you had an unacknowledged expectation attached.

"I'm allowed to *hope* we're a good match though, right?"

Yes, of course you are. The primary difference between a **hope** and an **expectation** is the attachment you have to the outcome. You may *hope* that you hit it off with your date, you enjoy the way they kiss, or you get to explore sexually together. If those things don't work out, it's okay to be bummed. If you had the *expectation* those things would happen, you may find your ego gets damaged when the chips don't fall exactly as you planned. This small mind shift between hope and expectation affects the emotional impact on everyone.

Expectations are grounded in rigidity. Hope is grounded in flexibility. Expectations are humorless. Hope can have a sense of surprise or humor. Expectations are about force. Hope is about acceptance.

Navigating Expectations

I like to use the "full disclosure" method to navigate both my and my partners' expectations. It allows me to point to what may be an easy misunderstanding and clarify it. I might say, "Full disclosure: I have an early meeting so I need to go home right after dinner," or, "Full disclosure: The host of the party is my ex, but it's chill." If your date says or does something that contradicts your expectation, try to point to it, right away:

"I have to be at the train station at nine."

"Oh, I thought we were going to the movies together."

> "Your portion comes out to $57.82."

> "I imagined you were treating tonight since I bought the theater tickets."

> "My buddies are on their way."

> "I wanted it to be just the two of us tonight."

True, this may derail some things. But unspoken and unmet expectations breed resentment. You can speak up and try to clarify or compromise, or you can stew silently and convince yourself they're a jerk. The first option, while more awkward up front, may save you a lot of frustration down the line.

When two people meet for the first time, there are going to be hiccups. If something feels ambiguous, address it and seek clarification. If you're wondering about something, it's possible they are, too. Correct the record where necessary, go with the flow when possible, and compromise where you can, but don't forget your absolute deal breakers. Those apply during all phases of relationships, from first dates to thirtieth anniversaries.

Don't underestimate the power of tone of voice. The style and tone with which you deliver awkward news or get clarity can make all the difference.

Consider this phrase: "Is this a date?"

Say it aloud like you're freaked out and accusing someone of tricking you.

Now say it like you're delighted to be spending time with a person.

See the difference? That change can be *everything* when getting to know someone. I'm not suggesting we all have to be classically trained actors ready to deliver a line eight different ways, but it's a good idea to pay attention to *how* you say things just as much as what you say.

If you lean in for a kiss and they pull away, one or both of you may have been misreading the other. That's not a huge deal, but it may warrant an apology and a request for clarity. Getting called out can be embarrassing. Chalk it up to more information, both about yourself and the connection between the two of you. Thank them for offering clarity, take responsibility for unclear communication if your expectation was erroneous, and use that information moving forward.

MANAGING DISAPPOINTMENT

Though less severe than rejection, disappointment can still sting like whoa. Disappointment usually occurs when someone or something fails to meet your expectations (whether reasonable or not). It's okay to feel sad, frustrated, or unappreciated.

Acknowledge your feelings and name them. Then, mine your expectations for unmet needs. Are you needing TLC and think a sleepover will give you that? Are you craving more one-on-one time, so these group hangs are hurting your feelings? Use this information to figure out how to meet these needs for yourself in other ways or make more specific requests. Source from multiple places wherever possible to avoid placing the brunt of your expectations on one single person or one single behavior.

You can't force people to act or feel a certain way. Nor can you force yourself to just *not* feel something. You *can* control how you act in a situation, however. So control what you can. Let the rest go.

Rejection

Sometimes you're gonna want someone who doesn't want you back. Sometimes people are gonna want you and you won't be interested. Welcome to the wonderful world of rejection.

Both being rejected and rejecting other people is hard. So hard that many folks come up with passive-aggressive, convoluted, and just lousy ways of avoiding it. Ghosting, sending out-of-left-field texts, stringing people along, or just flat-out lying are all ways people try to get out of having to take responsibility for their feelings.

It makes sense. Our culture puts a whole lot of value on sexual desire. When people take an interest in us, we're supposed to be flattered and humble, eager and open. But sex and relationships need to be two-way streets. When you run the odds, most of the time we're not on the same page as other folks. The better you can get at not taking it personally or overanalyzing the myriad of reasons why a person is telling you no, the happier everyone will be.

DELIVERING REJECTION

There are a million ways to say no, though some are clearer than others. "No" is a complete sentence. If someone offers you something, and you say no to them, that's a complete exchange. Many people have a hard time just saying the word by itself, especially if the asker hasn't crossed any boundaries, because it sounds too stern. In this case, folks often tack on the ever-lovely "thank you." The key is to be friendly but firm.

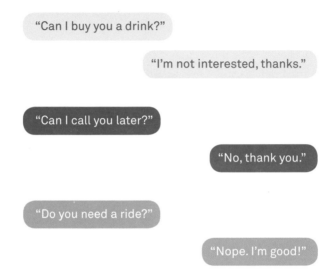

There's no need to hem and haw. In fact, the more you try to tack on excuses and add caveats, the more likely you may actually offend someone. You're allowed to add polite flourishes, but avoid equivocating or making excuses for your no. Here are a few other phrases that might work: "I'm noticing . . .," "I appreciate you taking the time to spend with me, but . . .," or "This has been enjoyable, but. . . ."

The key is to hold firm to your boundaries. You said no. Now the onus is on the other person to respectfully deal with that no. Sometimes people just don't understand things well the first time, but other, crappier people like to exploit indecisiveness or treat a no as a challenge. You can choose how you want to deal. If they keep pressing or don't hear you, you can state it again, or you can take pains to leave the situation. Sometimes you have to be diplomatic, but it's still best to be straightforward, for example, "I'm going to keep saying no. So you can waste both of our time or you can change the subject." If the person is pressing too hard and not taking your no for an answer, you can enlist help in the form of a friend or staff at the venue, or you can just get out of there and find a friendlier place to hang out.

Sometimes saying no is doing the other person a big favor. If your date does something inexcusable, like making racist jokes or treating the staff rudely, you are under no obligation to stick around. You can lecture them if you want to, or you can just thank them for their time and then hightail it out of there. Hopefully it'll be an opportunity for them to correct their behavior and speak with more compassion. Even for less shocking issues, telling someone "No thanks" can help let them off the hook. They can manage their disappointment, then be free to find a better fit.

Dating and sex can kick up our worst, most painful insecurities. While a simple "no" to a stranger at the bar is usually fine, if you've shared some intense moments with someone, odds are they deserve a little more tenderness. If you need to reject someone you've formed a significant bond with, like a long-term lover, jet on over to the Breakups section on page 233.

HANDLING REJECTION

When handling a rejection yourself, remember to take no for an answer. No *is* an answer, a perfectly good (if slightly painful) one. Just accept it, because no one owes you an explanation. Even if you had an amazing time. Even if you thought you'd get a regular thing going. Even if you made them come twelve times, they don't owe you an explanation. People are complicated. That's just how it is sometimes.

Instead of pressing them, thank the other person for speaking up. This is for *both* of you. It makes them feel like less of a jerk, but magically, for you, thanking a person can help you convince yourself they did you a favor. Why else would you be *thanking them*?! It really does work like a charm. By rejecting you, they gave you back your time and energy to direct to someone or something that actually wants and deserves it.

Baggage and Intersectionality

When you enter the wild world of casual sex, remember everyone's coming to the bedroom with a different mosaic of life experiences. Some people, based on their race, class, gender, sexual identity, and ability, will have mosaics that look different from yours. They may have been told things about their desirability, beauty, and potential based on those things.

You don't need to play therapist with *anyone*, but you *do* need to be a decent, compassionate person by acknowledging that everyone's got different cultural baggage.

Here's how to deal:

Don't take things personally. For example, if you're a man, and a woman is expressing hesitation about coming home with you, you can react in one of two ways: (1) get offended that she thinks you're a murderous rapist, or (2) assume she is protecting herself due to prior bad experiences and/or lessons she's learned growing up as a woman in society. The former reaction is a great way to develop resentment. The latter is a way to develop compassion. Which would you rather foster?

Thank people for speaking up. It's a big deal to ask for what you need to feel comfortable and safe—especially for people who are often told they're making shit up or being irrational. If someone tells you what they need, thank them, and see what you can do to make it happen.

Be aware of power dynamics. In every relationship there are power dynamics at work. One of you may have more money, a more stable job, a stronger capacity for communication, more life experience, more ease of mobility, a more loving home environment, and so on. You don't have to apologize for the things you have. You merely need to acknowledge that not everyone else has them. This is what people mean when they say, "Check your privilege." It doesn't mean you have to give up your belongings or dedicate your life to activism (but you can if that's your jam). It *does* mean it's good to note when you're making erroneous assumptions about how everyone else lives based on your own experience.

Risk and Power

If you're meeting people with the intention to have sex, it's helpful to be aware of your privileges and not take them for granted. Start by understanding the many ways in which these power dynamics can show up.

The following are some common social discrepancies between people. Note where you have challenges and where you have ease. Consider what other challenges people may have. More important, pay attention to things you haven't even thought of before! This stuff becomes really significant when you're choosing venues for dates or inviting people back to your place.

Mobility: The ability to navigate stairs, sit comfortably on barstools, or move through tight spaces all relate to mobility. What are your favorite date spots that may be inaccessible to other people?

Allergies/sensitivities: Perfumes, chemicals, animals, or foods can make people ill or trigger severe reactions. What venues do you frequent that have strong scents or allergens?

Money and class: Humans use a bunch of subtle and overt cues to indicate economic and social status, including manner of dress, accent, and lots of coded language. Some people may feel unsafe entering certain class-coded spaces because they may fear being ostracized or shamed. And of course, how much money you have determines what you can afford to do, and where you can afford to live or visit.

Housing: Do you own your home or do you rent? Is your rent stabilized? Do you rely on roommates/family to cover living expenses? Do you trust your landlord? Is your housing situation secure, or do you have to behave in a certain way to keep a roof over your head? If you lost your income tomorrow, how long until you wouldn't have a place to live? Everyone has a different housing situation that affects what they can afford and if they can bring people back to their place after a date.

Gender: Most spaces (in the whole damn world) are safer for men than they are for women. Most spaces (in the whole damn world!) are safer for cis people than they are for trans people. Certain spaces have gender rules that can make people feel unwelcome or unsafe.

Sexual orientation: Being visibly queer is still dangerous in many parts of the world. Biphobia is real, too, leading some bi people to feel unwelcome in queer spaces.

Race: It can be uncomfortable, scary, or even downright dangerous to be the odd one out in a room full of people who don't look like you. Historical racial inequities can make it hard for some folks to be themselves or relax around people of other races.

Health care access: If you get injured/sick, how likely are you to receive quality health care? This can limit date/kink activities. Can you access emergency contraception or abortion services, or prenatal care?

Passing privilege: Passing privilege often refers to trans people being able to "pass" as cis. How well you look like you "belong" somewhere. It can also apply to queer people passing as straight, people of color passing as white, or working class people passing as upper class, among others.

Language and accent: Some people are marked as "other" simply by the way they speak. Sometimes it can be a cute conversation starter, but in some cases it can be a big ol' glowing arrow pointing out they don't fit in.

Immigration status: Interactions with both law enforcement and every-day folks can be dicey for people with complicated immigration status.

Education: Advanced education more often indicates social status than it does intelligence. Many folks may feel ostracized for not having high school or college degrees.

Trauma/PTSD: Some people have serious emotional triggers and they need to take pains to avoid certain situations. For instance, fireworks can be triggering to veterans and people who grew up around gun violence.

Neurodiversity: We make lots of assumptions as to how an "average" human brain works. As with everything human, though, diversity is the rule, including how different people process information.

This is by no means an exhaustive list, and I'm sure you could come up with more ways in which social situations are more or less navigable based on indi-viduating factors.

Even if you aren't actively discriminated against for being the odd one out on any of these metrics, it can still create a mental burden. You may feel extra vigi-lant about maintaining your cover or trying hard to fit in. It can add an extra layer of complication or nervousness to a date or sexual interaction.

How to deal? Don't ignore difference. Take stock of the potential risk factors your date venue/activity presents and try to make them explicit. Let your date know you're open to their suggestions or needs. Consider your favorite date ven-ues and how they may not be accessible to everyone. Practice advocating for yourself and letting your date know what you'd need to feel comfortable. You're giving them the chance to win with you and also learning a whole lot about your compatibility.

Risk Aversion

We all move through the world with different challenges, and it's vital we understand how different people respond to **risk**.

The more privileges you have, the less risk-averse you have to be. If you're a legal citizen, it's less risky to drive above the speed limit. If you're white, it's less risky for you to interact with police. If you aren't relying on a full scholarship, it's less risky to cut class. If you don't have a uterus, it's less risky to have unprotected sex.

Humans make choices for a whole slew of reasons, and only some of those reasons may make sense to you. If someone seems fussy or "high maintenance," it may be because they're controlling for things that might not even show up on your radar. Give people the benefit of the doubt. It doesn't have to be some giant conversation. Just as I've gotten accustomed to asking dinner guests, "Any food restrictions?" before planning a menu, the more we can be aware of the issues other folks have that we don't, the better off everyone can be.

Here are some more examples to consider. Some people may:

→ Need to get a certain GPA to keep their scholarship so they can stay in school. So cutting class is out of the question.

→ Have had a traumatic experience with law enforcement. So anything that brings them in proximity to cops is terrifying.

→ Be working through addiction issues, making places with alcohol, tobacco, or drugs hard to enjoy.

→ Have a criminal record, which means they need to stay away from places where underage people are drinking.

→ Need to avoid loud or crowded places because of an emotional or physical disability or PTSD.

→ Stick to a rigorous medication schedule, making spontaneity difficult.

→ Have a chronic medical condition that can be exacerbated by STIs, making safer sex protocols *super* important.

→ Have a history that includes sexual violence, making some sexual acts or language quite scary.

None of these means you can't have hot, fun sexy-times with people who have different risk awareness than you. It just means it's a good idea to be sensitive to their needs and realize not everyone has the same comfort with risk-taking.

If you neglect to disclose something important to your date, you're not a bad person. You just probably have never encountered these issues before. Not every undisclosed privilege is a deal breaker or some sort of giant conversation. Just do your best to be sensitive to other people's needs. Once you become aware of individual challenges, you can front-load them into your conversations to give everyone the chance to be informed:

> "You wanna come back to my place? I have a cat and my roommates are all dudes, but they're cool."

There's no way you can know all the nuances of your partner's needs up front. Everything from triggers to preferences can be complex and hard to anticipate. The best way to navigate is to acknowledge the obvious power dynamics, offer opt-ins, and be open to other suggestions:

> "I rented a movie."

> "I don't do well with violent films."

> "Okay, how about we browse Netflix and find something we'd both like?"

If your date isn't forthright about their needs, you can still aim for flexible opt-ins:

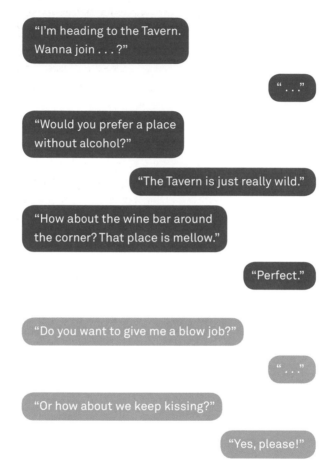

"I'm heading to the Tavern. Wanna join . . . ?"

" . . . "

"Would you prefer a place without alcohol?"

"The Tavern is just really wild."

"How about the wine bar around the corner? That place is mellow."

"Perfect."

"Do you want to give me a blow job?"

" . . . "

"Or how about we keep kissing?"

"Yes, please!"

See? None of these has to be a fraught conversation. They just give every-one an opportunity to advocate for themselves and opt in. In general, grace and flexibility are virtues. So if someone raises an issue, respect it and offer alternatives. If someone thinks it's sexy when you make all the plans, this can get a little trickier. Try asking if they have any preferences or restrictions at all, and then work from there.

If someone rejects you for a reason you don't understand, or asks for an accommodation that doesn't make sense to you, do your own research. While you may be able to ask the person in a sensitive way, the internet is often a bet-ter way to do research without expecting that person to be the oracle for your inquiry. Being aware of the complexities of humanity has an added benefit of raising your sexual cachet. Being more sensitive to people's experiences makes you better in bed, a more desirable partner, and a better person in general.

Gender Trouble

When I was younger, I broke a lot of hearts. See, I was a perfect product of my culture, which taught me boys only want one thing. So when I used boys for that one thing and then subsequently rejected them like bad organs, many of them ended up hurt. No one taught me boys have romantic feelings, just like girls, and they can have crushes and feel devoted, too. Meanwhile, lots of boys get taught that girls are fickle, fragile things. When we're upset, we're "crazy," and when we have requests, we're "needy." The stereotypes for both these genders are unfair and detrimental to good sex. The result is people don't talk to each other.

If you're LGBTQ+, don't think you get off scot-free. Many of us fall into the same trap of stereotyping our community, often still based on the feminine/masculine binary. Thus, femmes get called crazy, and butches have to act like studs. Gay tops have to be "masc," and only sissies are bottoms. Trans women are considered catty. Trans men are thought of as aggro.

One of the best things you can do when you catch yourself flippantly assigning a meaning to a partner's behavior based on often-arbitrary traits such as gender (or race or age) is to instead relate to them as *people*. Shocking, I know. Refrain from assuming you know their exact thought process and their next action based on their identity label.

Assumptions are boring. You essentially make up your mind about someone before you get a chance to know them. Where's the fun in that? Not every trans gal is femme. Not every genderqueer person is pansexual. Not every cis guy wants to fuck around. Not every trans dude used to identify as a lesbian. Not every straight gal is waiting for a wedding ring. These days, those stereotypes are becoming more and more antiquated, but many of us still have them entrenched in our minds, and we're coming up with new ones every day. So when someone tells us something true for them, we may be incredulous or surprised.

Sure, people change, and sometimes people lie about who they are. But it's still usually a better idea to take people at face value. In the famous words of Maya Angelou: "When someone shows you who they are, believe them the first time."

When I met my partner, he was with his boyfriend, so I assumed he was gay (and monogamous). It wasn't until he hit on me that I realized what was up. I was so confused, I almost didn't believe him when he said he wanted to kiss me. It hadn't even *occurred* to me he could be bi, because of my own assumptions about the prevalence of bisexual men.

Once I finally accepted he *was* bi, however, I had a hard time believing he'd want to be with someone like me: hairy-legged, heavily tattooed, dykey-looking me. Because I had *another* idea in my head that men didn't like women who looked like me.

If I had hewed to those stereotypes instead of taking him at his word, I could have missed out on the great love of my life!

On Labels

Sometimes you crave a kind of person you've never been with before. Maybe you're a lesbian who starts fantasizing about hairy chests and gruff voices. Maybe you're a straight guy who just has a thing for Chris Evans, he's a handsome dude, okay?! Or maybe you're a gal who's always been into blue-collar guys but something about that genderqueer librarian just makes you feel things.

Here's the big reveal: Yep, that happens. Welcome to the club.

Identity labels are just words. Language is a faulty, frail thing. The divisions between labels are mostly arbitrary and simply help our feeble human brains categorize shit. Yet most of the planet spends their lives trying to figure out who is _____ enough to be a part of their team. The fact is most of us will never measure up to every standard. We're not skinny enough, rich enough, Black enough, queer enough, radical enough, trans enough, multi-ethnic enough, well-read enough, blah dee fucking blah.

Labels can be helpful, I'll admit. They're great for dating profiles and nutritional information. They can help you find a community and plant your garden. When you start using labels as *prescriptive* rather than *descriptive*, though, you're on shaky ground. Remember: You have control over how you want to interpret or use a word. You define your identity. It doesn't define you. If a label works for a while and then stops working as well, you can change it. If the labels you use change meaning based on your context, you can change them or double-down on your choice. If following your inner sense of rightness takes you down a gender or orientation path that frightens you, you get to choose how far you travel.

In the thirty-eight years I've been on this planet, I've gone from bi to lesbian to queer to monogamous to polyamorous to vanilla to kinky to cis to gender-indifferent to whatever the fuck. And I've still got a lot of living left to do. Identities are living things. In the '90s, no one called themselves "cis." In the '80s, "queer" was mainly a slur. Who knows what new identities will blossom in the future?

Many people change their sexual identities at least once in their lives. Sometimes it's because circumstances change (their partner decides to change their gender, perhaps, or they move to a new part of the world that has a different understanding of certain words). Sometimes a person claims a new identity because the context of the word shifts. Sometimes it's because they discover a new word that fits better. Changing your identity can be a great choice. Sometimes doing it twelve times is the right thing to do. Your parents might roll their eyes, but your identity isn't about them, or anyone. It's how you relate to yourself.

PRO TIP

Even if you're flexible or experimenting with your gender or identity, that doesn't mean your potential playmate is. Suggesting anyone is "just going through a phase" or "doing it wrong" is condescending. Likewise suggesting a straight girl just "hasn't been with the right woman yet" or a monogamous person is a tool of the patriarchy or whatever, is bullshit.

My overarching advice? Follow love. Trust your inner sense of rightness. You get to choose how you show up for every relationship that presents itself. You'll likely be best served by following a choice that leads to more love, not less. If you head toward rightness and love, you'll likely make the right steps, or at least you'll be able to tell where the right steps are.

Consent and Communication

Like it or not, when you get it on with people, you're going to have to discuss it. Telepathy isn't real. You're responsible for communicating your likes, dislikes, boundaries, and desires with your partners. I know this can be tough. I've been teaching sex ed for over ten years now and I still have a hard time speaking up sometimes.

The good news is that there's *plenty* to like about clear communication. It means you care about your partner's pleasure, comfort, and emotional state. It sets you up to win, and can help you rock worlds. The people who say it isn't "organic" are simply full of shit. What's *not* organic is getting stuck in your own head because you're lost or triggered or picking up ambiguous signals—or no signals at all.

Consent

Presumably (hopefully), you're reading this book at least in part because you're trying to figure out this whole "consent" thing.

Well, good, because I have got *a lot* to say about it.

Some of it may be along the lines you'd expect, like, "Hey, don't rape people."

Some of it may be a little . . . surprising. My thoughts are my own, and I invite you to do some serious thinking on where you stand on this stuff yourself. Our cultural understandings of consent are changing rapidly and intensely. So let's dive, face-first, into the wild world of **consent**.

"Consent" can feel like a scary word. It's so often associated with horrifying nonconsensual situations, making it difficult to discuss in any way that feels remotely sexy. But it's a skill you can learn like any other and it's a necessary concept to grok. When it's done well, it's super sexy.

The bar for literal consent is actually set pretty low. All it means is everyone is agreeing to the activity. You can get basic consent by simply asking if someone wants to do something and then waiting for them to say yes.

This low bar is just a start, so let's consider two upgrades:

Informed consent means everyone's on the same page and crystal clear. It means deconstructing euphemisms and discussing expectations. For example, if you consent to "watersports" with me, you might be disappointed when I don't show up with a jet ski.

Enthusiastic consent means not only agreement, but genuine enthusiasm for the proposed activity. Enthusiasm mitigates issues of bullying, coercion, intoxication, and peer pressure.

If negotiating sex is like choosing a restaurant, enthusiastic and informed consent is "China Grove? I love that place!" or "I've been meaning to try that place!" or "Yes, but I'm allergic to shrimp, so please don't order that." Enthusiastic, informed consent is *not*, "If it's really important to you" or "I don't know what the food is."

If the concept is still daunting to you, let's take it back to the root of the word. Essentially, consent is the practice of *consensus*. It means everyone gets a vote, and everyone's vote matters equally. A lack of consensus means the proposition won't move forward.

CONSENT IS . . .

→ **Consensus.**
All parties must agree on the activity.

→ **Revocable.**
Anyone is allowed to change their mind at any point, even midway into an activity.

→ **Respect.**
It's a way for everyone to feel safe and appreciated.

→ **Collaborative.**
It's an opportunity to use your voice and discuss likes and dislikes.

→ **Informational.**
It's an opportunity to learn about your partner. You may have no problem speaking up in the moment or getting yourself out of a situation you don't want to be in. But not everyone's like that.

→ **Revolutionary.**
We're living through an intense time when we're deconstructing the ways in which gender, sexuality, and power intersect. By demonstrating care and interest in the complexities of the human sexual experience, we're creating safer and more resilient communities and cultures. You can be a part of this sex culture revolution by investing your energy in this conversation.

The Limits of
Enthusiastic Consent

These days it's hip to talk about enthusiastic consent as though it's the magic bullet against the monster of sexual assault. It's true that enthusiastic consent is an effective tool to encourage people to make sure everyone involved is having a good time. However, enthusiastic consent has its limits and can falter under scrutiny. This is because there are many reasons for having sex, and being SUPER-DUPER EXCITED TO is really only one of those reasons.

If you've ever been to a twelve-step meeting, you know that varieties such as Alcoholics or Narcotics Anonymous encourage abstinence. That is, the ideal outcome of AA is that alcoholics never touch booze again. Never mind the fact that some problem drinkers may well be capable of developing a healthy relationship with alcohol. Because of the huge number of people seeking help from the program, however, the easiest way to help *the most people at once* is by encouraging hardline abstinence. In other twelve-step programs such as Overeaters Anonymous, you can't just tell people to quit food. They have to take a more nuanced approach, teaching people to develop healthy habits and improve their overall relationship with food.

Enthusiastic consent is the AA equivalent of consent models. It's a strict bar, but it likely helps the most people. Meanwhile, a more complete understanding of sexual consent may benefit from more of an OA model, wherein we teach people to listen to their bodies and make good choices.

Here are some situations when enthusiastic consent can miss the whole truth:

→ When you're not sure if you'll like something but want to try it anyway.

→ When you're using sex to process heavy emotions, like grief or trauma.

→ When you're in the closet and/or processing sexual shame.

→ When you're doing sex work.

→ When you're trying to get pregnant.

→ When you're super-duper nervous.

→ When you're having sex to make your partner happy.

→ When you're having sex to regulate your neurochemistry (as a distraction or fucking yourself into a better mood).

→ When you started off enthusiastic but lost your verve and decided to stick with it anyway.

→ When you started off *un*enthusiastic but knew eventually your joy would catch up.

In these scenarios you may find enthusiasm in some respects but not all. For example, you may be enthusiastic about seeing a sex work client so you can pay your rent. Or you may be enthusiastic about making your partner feel good even if the sex itself is "meh." Or you may really want to make a baby even though it's gonna take some effort to "get there" emotionally.

I don't think it's fair to say, as is common in some sex ed circles, that anything less than a "Hell yes!" is a no. The key is, as always, to be mindful and communicative about it. If you're less than over-the-moon about the sex you're having, that's fine. But that's *your* decision to make for yourself, not someone else's decision to make for you. And be aware that opting in to less-than-enthusiastic sex can hurt your partner's feelings, too. If you think it's appropriate to make the dynamic explicit, do it.

If you're having sex because you think that's the only way you can be close to someone you like, take a moment to interrogate that assumption. Maybe you could have just as much fun exploring sensual touch instead of sexual touch, or doing something intimate (like having a deep conversation) that doesn't involve touch at all.

If your partner doesn't seem very enthusiastic, pause and check in. A person can choose to engage in nonenthusiastic sex, but that doesn't mean everyone has to. Let's think of consent, and sex in general, as collaborative. Rather than enthusiasm, which puts the onus on the participants to generate a *feeling*, collaboration requires everyone to bring something to the table, but those things don't have to be identical.

For example:

→ You want sex and I want money.

→ You want to get pregnant and I want to help.

→ You want to process some heavy feelings and I want to practice my flogging technique.

→ You want to forget about your ex for an hour and I want to eat pussy.

To make this work, you must **take responsibility for your choices**. Name them. Know what you're looking for and why. Once you've decided what you're interested in, find how it fits into what the other person is up for. If there's no middle ground to be found, honor their choices, thank them for their time, and move on. You don't get to make up other people's minds for them. Similarly, you also don't have to tolerate people's choices that violate your desires and boundaries.

There are infinite combinations of the *why* we have sex. The pleasure of sex is often the most common reason, but it's not the *only* one. Be forthright, honest, and respectful about your reasons and see if the other person buys in. You may be surprised about how many valid places people can meet that are about more than just "WHEEEE SEX!"

Emotional Consent

When we talk about consent, the conversation is often only about the sex itself. But consent starts well before that, and includes emotional well-being. For instance, if someone is having sex with me based on the idea that I really, really like them and now we're dating, *but* I'm hooking up with them based on the idea we're both just feeling the vibe of the night and there is no relationship forming, guess what's missing? *Informed* consent! I did not inform them of my desires and neither did they! Even if no one feels *violated* afterward, per se (though one certainly could), there are still likely to be hurt feelings going around that could have been avoided with clear communication.

So, when things start moving into the sexual realm, as well as communicating the basic physical consent stuff, also communicate your *emotional* needs.

"Want to go back to my place?"

"I do. But I want to know if you'd like to go out sometime, like on a date."

"I'm not available for that right now. I'm just looking for some casual fun."

"Maybe we shouldn't, then. I think it'll just make me sad."

"Can I go down on you?"

"I want you to, but I only let people I'm monogamous with do that."

"Well, you're the only person I'm seeing right now, and I like it that way."

"Really? Let's discuss this, because I'd really like to be your sweetie."

"I'd like that, too."

The Art of the Check In

I go to lots of sex parties. I host them, too. If you've never been in a room where dozens of people are having all sorts of extraordinary sex while others watch and snack and cuddle, I'm going to let you in on a secret: there's a *lot* of negotiation. Many orgies have between forty-five minutes and two hours of sharing in a circle before the sex even starts. We talk about STI status, pronouns, likes/dislikes, limits, and more. We talk about what we want so people can give it to us. We talk about what we don't want so people know what to avoid. Even without a welcome circle, at a good sex party there is always a *ton* of talking. So if a room full of freaky-ass freaks can talk at length and still have a grand ol' time, you can, too.

Checking in saves you emotional paperwork the next day. "Just going with it" can feel good in the moment, but in the cold light of day, you may have second thoughts. Much day-after drama could be mitigated by checking in before, during, and after sex. It also ensures you get what you actually want. Too often we defer to what we *think* our partner wants instead of asking for what we want. This creates sex where both people are doing what they think the other one wants instead of actually talking about it.

Checking in also helps you get repeat business. If your partner feels respected and heard, they're more likely to want to see you again. If they feel as though you took good care of them in bed, they may even recommend you to their friends. Have you ever gotten laid on recommendation before? I have. It's fucking awesome.

Remember there's no such thing as "just knowing." There is only "getting so used to one act you go on autopilot." This may be fine if you have a string of sex partners who all like the exact same thing, but as soon as you work that move on someone who doesn't like it, you're in trouble.

The easiest part about checking in *before* sex is you can do it whenever: like over dessert, walking home from the movies, or making out at the front door. Even if you've been seeing someone for a while, it's never too late to check in about this stuff. You can always learn more about your partner and their body.

> Naomi and I liked to go to yoga class on dates and then check in while showering together afterward. We'd scrub each other's backs and discuss what we'd like to explore that night and any relevant things that may have happened since our last date. By the time we were done, we were squeaky clean and ready to get down to business.

Remember "You 101" back on page 18? Now is the time when it comes in really handy! That's the stuff to frontload before sexy-time. As a brief refresher, You 101 is:

→ Words you like and words you don't

→ STI status and safer sex protocols

→ Relationship status and boundaries

→ No Zones and boundaries

→ Likes and turn-ons

→ Any other quirks you want them to know

Think of You 101 as your preflight checklist—a crash course into the basics of you. Beyond those basics, there are few other things to consider when negotiating a roll in the hay. First, lead with the scary stuff. Nursing a broken heart? Inexperienced but eager? Dealing with chronic pain? To the best of your ability, it's a great idea to front-load all the stuff you think will scare someone away. The ones who stick around are the ones you want anyway.

Next, address your hopes. This is a biggie. What do you want to get out of the experience? This can be specific to the person or the interaction. Want to practice your blow job technique? Want to try some new positions with an enthusiastic partner? Just want to get eaten out for thirty relaxing minutes? Whatever it is, say so. This is part of consent. Let your potential partner opt in with full awareness.

Disclosure

Need to have a bigger talk than just "I have a latex allergy"? Try having the conversation *before* you get to the bedroom. Over dinner, on a walk, or on a long drive can all be great times to broach the subject. If you have something big to share but don't know how to do it, here's an excellent formula to try. (I'm swiping this from relationship genius, and my partner, Reid Mihalko. Thanks, babe!)

ReidAboutSex's Difficult Conversation Formula

1 I have something to tell you.

2 Here's what I'm afraid will happen when I tell you . . .

3 Here's what I want to have happen . . .

4 Here's what I have to tell you . . .

Let's see some examples:

> "I have something to tell you. I haven't told you because I don't want to hurt you. What I want is that we can continue on as friends and stay in each other's lives. So what I have to tell you is I'm falling for someone and we want to be monogamous."

> "Before our date, I want you to know something. I haven't told you because I've been rejected for it before and I really like you. I want to still see you, because I'm still 100 percent the person you think I am. So I need you to know I'm trans."

The formula works for all sorts of situations. I use it for big and small things in my relationships—everything from coming clean about a white lie to having a Serious Talk About the Future of Us. If you're afraid of sharing something with a lover, consider why. If you're actually concerned for your safety if you disclose something, consider if you want to go to bed with this person at all. Meanwhile, if you're afraid of rejection or your partner freaking out, there are ways to deal.

→ Try the Difficult Conversation Formula.

→ Have the talk when you both aren't naked and entwined.

→ Accept the possibility that your partner may indeed freak out a little bit. Most people don't handle new information well, and few of us love hearing the words "Can we talk?" Allow your partner time to process the information. They may come around once they've had a chance to sit it with it for a while.

→ If you being honest and straightforward about something important to you freaks out your partner, consider the fact they just saved you lots of emotional baggage down the road. Do you really want to date/sleep with/fall for someone who can't handle something true and real for you? Sure, it may not make it any less sucky, and you may have really liked that person. Being vulnerable by disclosing some of your Real Shit™ can open you up to hurt and rejection. But it's better to be rejected for who you are than accepted for who you aren't.

HEARING DISCLOSURES

The complexity and diversity of the human experience means you cannot control for every variable. You can, however, minimize grief by establishing yourself as a compassionate person. Nearly everyone has something they're afraid to share, whether it's an identity, a desire, an aversion, or a body issue. The more people you get to know in both sexual and nonsexual environments, the more adept you can be at dealing with complex human situations.

The key is not to force, or even encourage, anyone to disclose intimate details about themselves. Rather, help the person feel safe to share with minimal fear by being a beacon of empathy for them. Sometimes you can set the stage by disclosing some of your own stuff up front.

Eradicate ableist, racist, misogynistic, and other bigoted speech and thinking from your life. Learn how to handle new information with grace and gratitude. Let people know they're safe to share the scary stuff with you. This doesn't mean you'll always get it perfect or people will always speak up, but keep trying. The results are worth it.

Boundaries

Boundaries are standards a person sets to delineate how they want to be treated and how they want to interact with the world. We all have boundaries for touch, emotional intimacy, time, and any other human interaction. Each one is different and they usually change based on the familiarity between people. (My touch boundaries with my partner, for instance, are quite different from my touch boundaries with my mechanic.) Some of us are good at setting and maintaining our boundaries. Others, especially those with codependency issues, really aren't. When you date and sleep with people, you tend to get a crash course in how other people maintain their boundaries.

Ideal boundaries are strong, flexible (not to be mistaken for permeable), and clearly articulated. When you understand your boundaries, it's easier to negotiate sex and assert your needs and wants. When you articulate your boundaries and invite your partner to do the same, sex becomes a collaboration rather than a transaction. Sex is not the handshake after the haggle. You're deciding, *together*, what you want to do and create, *together*.

The key, though, is to articulate your boundaries. Because boundaries are so individualized, it's impossible to know what boundaries a person has until you discuss them. If you don't state your boundaries, your partner can't honor them. When your boundaries are flexible and healthy, it's easier to articulate and protect them. If you find yourself getting rocked when anyone accidentally hits even a minor boundary, if you retreat or get angry, or if you get feedback that you give off mixed signals, you may need to do some work on shoring up self-confidence and communication skills.

I like to think of boundaries in intimate relationships as a Venn diagram. I'm circle A, you're circle B, and where those circles overlap is the relationship.

Some Venn diagrams have little to no overlap (and therefore little to no relationship) and some are so overlapped they look like one circle (enmeshment, as can happen in codependent relationships). Regardless of how your Venn diagram with a partner may look, these boundaries define intimacy opportunities.

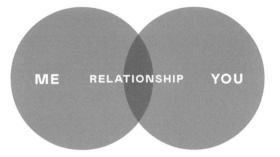

This diagram is helpful because it shows not only what's outside the boundaries but what is *inside*. See, some folks have a mistaken notion that boundaries are only what you *don't* want. But they're also what you *do*. Boundaries give you the chance to ask for what you want and to see where you and your partner overlap.

BOUNDARIES IN BED

The best thing you can do for your sex life is to expand the idea of what counts as sex. Sex doesn't have to look one way—in fact, it rarely looks the same way twice! There's no reason why you can't have a hot and fulfilling romp with someone even if certain sex acts aren't on the table. When you expand your repertoire of sex acts and pleasurable experiences, the number of people you can connect with *and* the ways you can connect with them increase exponentially.

Over my career as a slutty slut slut, I've had the privilege of working within a whole bunch of boundaries. Sometimes penetrative sex is off the table, sometimes oral is the no-go, and sometimes no genital touch is the rule of the day. Why any of my partners choose to draw those boundaries is entirely up to them. All I have to decide is whether or not I can hang with the boundaries they set. Sometimes you'll find you'd rather not play by the defined rules. That's fine; you can always take your toys and go home. Other times, you may find constraint inspires creativity, and you can explore awesome new ways to have fun even if your go-to activities aren't on the menu.

One of the best ways to figure out how to have a fulfilling experience within constraints is by considering how you'd each like to *feel*. Want to feel cared for? Spent? Sexy as fuck? If you have a sense of what you're going for, you can consider multiple ways of arriving there, which you can then turn into actionable, specific requests. If you want to feel objectified, why not give your partner a lap dance? If you want to feel ravaged, consider wrestling, whether or not genital touch is involved. One of the best parts of partnered sexual play is figuring out how to cocreate a mutually fulfilling experience. So consider boundaries as gifts instead of obstacles, and you may be amazed by what you come up with.

Magic Words

Okay, so they're interested. You're interested. Now what? If you're like me, usually an awkward moment or two. I'm going to teach you one of the best phrases in the world of sex-having. It's almost magic how well it works. I know firsthand, because it's another thing I learned from my partner, Reid Mihalko, and it's the reason why we got together in the first place. Okay, here it is:

> "I have an idea!"

Not what you were expecting, is it? But those four little words pack a punch! Why?

→ **It breaks the ice.** One of the hardest things to do after establishing mutual interest is actually getting the groove going. Eventually you have to kiss, or embrace, or start taking off clothes. "I have an idea" is a great way to initiate this.

→ **It's consent-based.** You're not telling the other person what to do. You're just issuing an invitation.

→ **It invites feedback.** After you share your idea, you can invite the other person to comment on the idea, whether it interests them or not.

→ **It's open-ended.** The idea can just get things going. After breaking the seal, odds are you'll both be more comfortable sharing ideas.

→ **It's a little silly.** Silly can be good, especially when getting with new people. Silly is friendly, inviting, and safe. So try being a little silly by announcing "I have an idea!" You may be surprised by the results.

Let's see it in action:

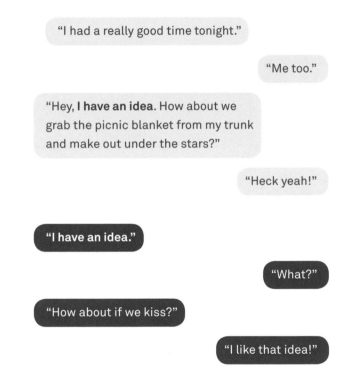

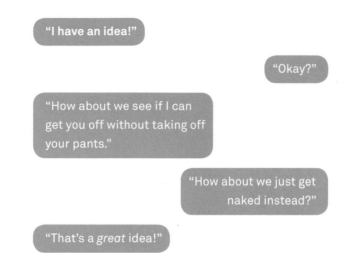

"I have an idea!"

"Okay?"

"How about we see if I can get you off without taking off your pants."

"How about we just get naked instead?"

"That's a *great* idea!"

The key to this formula is that once everyone agrees to the idea, you *initiate the thing*. Otherwise the awkward moment will come back and you have to come up with another idea. Be sure to deploy "I have an idea" only after you've established there's an erotic connection. As with anything, maintain flexibility and don't get too attached to your first idea. Be open to alternative suggestions and find that opt-in.

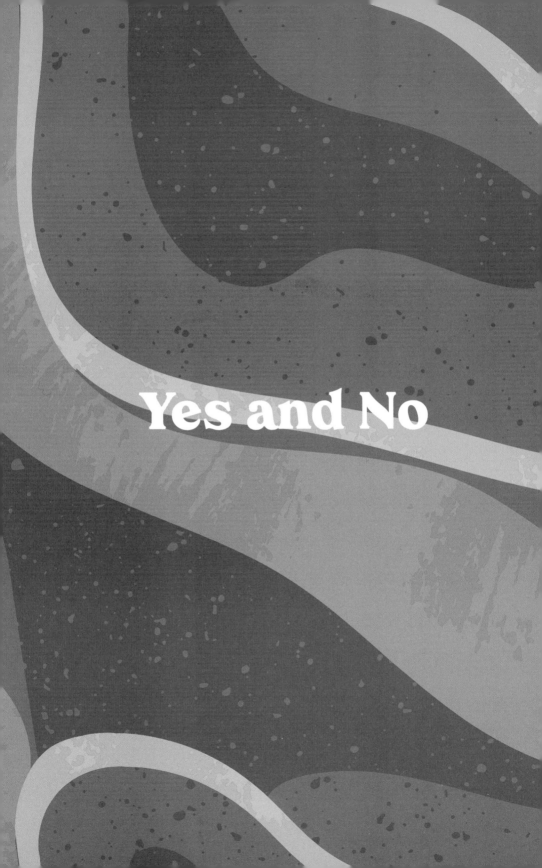

Yes and No

Some of us have a hard time saying no. Maybe it's society's fault. Maybe you were raised to be compliant. Maybe you're just a polite person and you don't like hurting people's feelings.

The thing is, if we can't say "no" in totally benign and low-stakes environments, how the hell can we expect to say it when sexy-times are imminent? It's like learning how to open a parachute once you've already leapt out of the plane. If you have a hard time saying no, I want you to practice as much as possible over the next twenty-four hours. Friends asking for favors, panhandlers asking for a quarter, strangers asking for a chair in a cafe: tell them all no.

You will likely feel like a bad person. You may feel guilt, shame, the pressure of privilege, and the anxiety of letting everyone down. GOOD. DO IT ANYWAY. You don't have to do it in a cruel way. A no with a smile can usually soften the blow. If you're *really* scared, try "Sorry, no." Don't go any further than that. It *should* feel hard and weird. That's the point. Saying "no" is like a muscle. Once it's properly bulked up, you can use it far more regularly than before, so taking it into the bedroom should become a breeze.

The Four Principles of No

1   **"No" is a complete sentence.**
    You don't have to justify it, explain it, or apologize for it. No is liberating for everyone involved. By telling someone no, you've given them permission to pursue something or someone else.

2   **Get good at saying no.**
    Every interaction could do with a few more no's. Especially from the feminine types. We're usually taught to be accommodating, friendly, pliant, and gracious at all times. Some of us take on that messaging more than others.

3   **If you want to get good at everything from flirting to sex to long-term relationships, get okay with hearing no.**
    You'll hear it plenty. It won't kill you. Most of the time, no isn't about you. It's because the object of your desire is taken, not into your flavor, or just not in the mood. The better you can get at not taking it

personally or overanalyzing the array of reasons why a person is telling you no, the happier everyone will be. Even when it *is* about you, a person telling you no is doing you a favor. A cold no is way better than a begrudging yes in terms of safety, self-care, and emotional paperwork.

4   **Learn what no *feels* like just as much as what it *looks* like.**
Many of us have a good intuition with no. Something just feels icky about the situation, or flee-worthy, or just anti-fun. The key is to make the connection between the feeling and the voice. When you know what no feels like in your own body, you almost always get better at noticing it in other people. This is a good thing. So listen to your inner voice and then articulate it, even if that means ending a date prematurely.

Understanding Soft No's

A **soft no** is any sort of response that is supposed to *mean* no, without actually using that word. You've probably heard "Maybe later," "Eh, I don't know," or "I wish I could" at some point—and you've probably said them, too. Soft no's are coded language meant to soften the perceived harshness of the simple word no. They are most often deployed in interactions with built-in power differentials. For example, if your boss says, "Can you stay late to do inventory tonight?," you may respond with something like, "I'm working a double-shift tomorrow." That's a soft no. You're trying to put the onus on your boss to assume what you mean, which in this case, is no. But, because they're your boss, you can't just say no, so you explain why you don't want to in a passive way. A soft no could be absolutely true or it could be a white lie. Either way, the point is the same: to say no without saying no.

People also do it in flirting and dating all the time:

"May I join you?"

"I'm waiting for a friend."

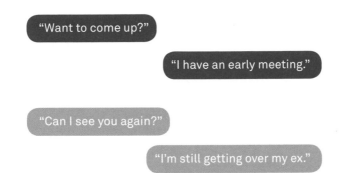

"Want to come up?"

"I have an early meeting."

"Can I see you again?"

"I'm still getting over my ex."

Soft no's often come from a person not feeling comfortable freely saying no. Many people who've had shitty interactions in the past will deploy them as a means of protecting themselves. It's frequently a strategy to avoid being hurt by people who can't handle rejection (or people, like your boss, who you would be unwise to reject directly).

Just because it's an entrenched strategy, doesn't mean soft no's don't cause problems. For instance, none of the previous examples give a clear response and let the asker off the hook. Instead, they invite confusion or more questions. A soft no puts the burden on the asker to read between the lines and interpret your intended meaning. You may think "I'm still getting over my ex" is an obvious no. But it could also mean, "Sure! I need to distract myself from my heartache!" or "I'm new to the dating world so let's take it slow." When it comes to sex, the most important takeaway is to identify when you're getting a soft no and treat it like it's a forthright no. If you're confused, politely ask for clarity. For example:

"May I join you?"

"I'm waiting for a friend."

"Would you like to wait alone or would you prefer company?"

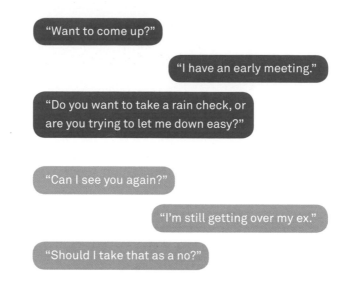

"Want to come up?"

"I have an early meeting."

"Do you want to take a rain check, or are you trying to let me down easy?"

"Can I see you again?"

"I'm still getting over my ex."

"Should I take that as a no?"

Persistence can create creepiness. So get clarity, but don't belabor the issue. A follow-up question that truly gives the other person the option of saying no without offense is a good way to make sure everyone is on the same page and feels free to use their words without negative repercussions.

GENDER AND "NO"

Many of us women and femme-types have been taught that men are unsafe. We may have been taught by female elders hoping to spare us some of the pain they've experienced. We may have been taught by men themselves, when they've hurt, threatened, or abused us. Or we just may learn it passively from the world at large. Many of us get that message starting young. Unfortunately, part of that message is, when men hurt us, it's our fault, period.

Sometimes it seems as if there are daily news stories of women who reject a man, even in a polite, docile manner, and are hurt or even killed for it. True, there are far more men who accept no and move on than there are men who lash out. However, these stories can cut us to the quick. We become afraid that the otherwise nice guy is going to snap. A lifetime of cautionary tales and bad experiences may have left us frightened and unwilling to trust our instincts. Try to hold space in your heart for this concept: Women and femmes are raised to be afraid of men. It may help you understand why so often we use a soft no instead of a true one.

This messaging runs so deep that women and femmes often deploy soft no's even with men we love and trust, and it takes practice to break the habit. Menfolk, please try to be patient with us. Ask clarifying questions if you need to and let us know you're one of the good ones by accepting our no's with grace and appreciation. Help us all get better at asserting ourselves and feeling safe doing so.

UPGRADING YOUR SOFT NO'S

It's pretty unfair to expect *unclear* language to be interpreted clearly. The onus is on all of us to communicate with as much clarity and integrity as possible. This is particularly true when it comes to a *very* common type of sexy-time communication: negotiation. Let's take a look at an example:

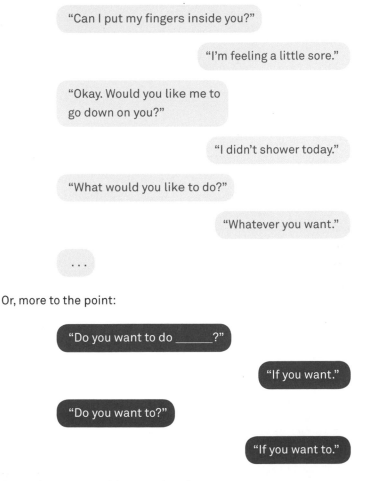

"Can I put my fingers inside you?"

"I'm feeling a little sore."

"Okay. Would you like me to go down on you?"

"I didn't shower today."

"What would you like to do?"

"Whatever you want."

. . .

Or, more to the point:

"Do you want to do _____?"

"If you want."

"Do you want to?"

"If you want to."

Damn, I got annoyed just writing that.

This kind of conversation happens *a lot*. Here's the thing, though: Can you tell what Person B actually wants? Do they want to be there? Are they feeling shy and need a little help relaxing? Or are they trying to get out of a situation they don't want to be in? This is one place where enthusiastic consent can be helpful, but it's not the whole story.

The sexual ideal is that we all have clarity of desire and facility with language, but most of us don't hit the ideal even a little bit. In the enthusiastic consent model, Person B doesn't seem too excited, so consent isn't possible. But it's also possible Person B is nervous because they *really* like Person A. Or they've internalized some sexual shame so making requests is scary. Or they're new to a certain kind of activity and genuinely don't know what they like.

If you find yourself in this position as Person A, *pull way back and check in*. If things are feeling hot and heavy but you're getting ambiguous signals, the best thing you can do is dial down the energy and have a clearheaded conversation. Sure, some of the wind may leave your collective sails, but it's better than getting stuck in your head about whether or not everyone's enjoying themselves. Here are some ways to broach the subject in a way that prevents hurt feelings:

"Hey, I'm getting some mixed signals. Can you let me know how you're feeling right now?"

"I'm really into being of service. Can you let me know what you like so I can make you feel good?"

"I feel like the energy just shifted. Is there something you want to discuss?"

"Maybe it's because I like you, but I'm feeling a little shy and awkward right now. Can you let me know how you're feeling?"

In these examples, the asker is taking on the responsibility to better understand their partner's needs. They noticed they needed more information and asked for it. It's not about forcing someone to decide on the spot what they want, but rather inviting them to offer clarity. There's nothing wrong with telling someone you need clearer signals to feel good about something. As with most human interactions, ignoring your instincts when things feel off causes more problems than pointing out the disconnect in the first place.

Remember, clear consent doesn't just protect the person who's receiving touch, but everyone involved. So if you don't feel good about the answers you're receiving, protect yourself by pulling back and potentially calling it quits. Once the clothes are back on and the heart rates have calmed, you may be able to have a clearer conversation about hopes and desires.

ACTIVE LISTENING

One of the quickest ways you can up your consent game is by developing your ability to listen to your partner, not only the words they say, but the way their body and energy communicate. When you touch your partner, do they recoil or soften beneath your fingers? When you look at them, do they avoid your gaze or meet it? When they answer your question, do they sound certain or hedging?

Active listening can help you decode mixed signals or press the brakes when you're not sure how things are going. Why is this important? Well, just like some people have learned to use soft no's to soften rejection, some folks also will say yes when they *don't* mean yes. They may even offer things they don't actually want to do because it feels easier than saying "Nah." This is a dangerous but unfortunately common form of muddy communication that can create agony for everyone involved. Practice listening to the words *and* the energy behind the words. Look for clarity, certainty, and connection in their body language and voice.

Embodied Yes & No

Some of us don't have a problem saying no—we're worse at saying yes! Yes can make us feel slutty or anxious or unsure of the next step. So, to get to the bottom of your feelings around saying yes, let's play a game. I'm going to state some assertions, and you're going to repeat them out loud or clearly in your head. With each one, feel the reaction in your body. *Take your time*, and don't move on until you've gotten a palpable sense of your reaction to each statement. Ready?

→ I am a woman.

→ I am straight.

→ I hate cats.

→ I love my father.

→ I believe in God.

→ Meat is delicious.

→ I have a great body.

→ Sex is pointless.

How was that for you? It's likely not all of these phrases pulled on your inner knowing, but maybe some of them did. Did any of them feel like lies? If you disagreed with any of them, what did it feel like? Was it a slightly repellent feeling? Was there a big energy to it? Did it make you feel alert or gross or frustrated or angry? What about things that felt true? What did that feel like? Exciting? Warm? Curious? Obvious?

Getting a sense of what yes and no feel like in your body can help you along when you're not sure what you're feeling. It can also help you speak up when something doesn't feel right. The goal is to get to a place where it's as easy to answer a question about sex as it is about whether you prefer cats or dogs. So let's try this again, now with more sexually charged questions. Again, repeat them out loud as though they are true statements, and feel into the answer before moving on.

→ I enjoy pain.

→ I want to tie people up.

→ I want to be anally penetrated.

→ I'm aroused by hard cocks.

→ I want to eat pussy.

→ I want to be the center of a gang bang.

How was that? It's possible you felt a little disgust response at some point. Again, that's fine. It's possible you found a hard no. It's also possible you found a well of arousal you think you're *supposed* to be disgusted by. Note it, but don't worry too much about it. It's all just information. It's also possible you found something that was a full-on yes. Feel into that yes and remember what it feels and sounds like. The better you get at hearing your Embodied Yes and Embodied No, the easier it gets to speak up on your way into bed and in bed.

Let's play with some more fill-in-the-blanks. We'll start mellow:

I love to feel _____ (a texture or sensation) _____

I want to try _____ (something sensual) _____

I'd love to explore _____ (a new activity) _____

Again, practice saying these aloud and with verve and enthusiasm.

Now, let's ramp it up:

I love _____ (sex act) _____

I want to try _____ (something sexual) _____

I'd love to explore _____ (yep, more sex) _____

Did you feel a little nervous? That's cool. Again, this takes practice. Practice asserting your desires in all aspects of your life. You'll likely get lots of positive reinforcement. In our daily lives, many of us are looking to one another for cues of how to proceed. If you're the one suggesting the movie or the next destination, you may find many people are relieved to let you call the shots for a little while.

Asking for What You Want

Asking for what you want is an essential part of a healthy relationship. If you don't want anything from a person, you don't have a relationship with them. You may have learned young that wanting things is a one-way ticket to disappointment town. You may have been shamed for having needs or making requests. Now, you may be so afraid of being told no, you don't even bother asking. Nevertheless, if you can't ask for what you want, your partner can't give it to you.

Good requests are **specific** ("I'd like to take you to dinner this weekend"), **actionable** ("Could you tell me what you like about me?"), and **relevant to the relationship** ("Can we use my vibrator together tonight?"). Try to upgrade feelings-based requests ("I want to feel loved") into something specific and actionable ("I want to go away for the weekend with you"). Avoid focusing on requests solely within your control ("I want to get to work on time tomorrow"). Instead, reframe them in a way that gives your partner some control by, say, asking them to make you coffee in the morning.

If you're not asking for what you want because you're afraid of rejection, do some work on your self-confidence (see page 39). Meanwhile, if you genuinely don't know what you want, it's time to do some homework. But before you do, communicate that with your partner(s), too. Insisting you "don't want anything" from someone comes across to most people as rejection, not comfort. If you don't know what you want from them, say so. It'll give them reassurance you actually want them in your life.

Try this: Send a text to a friend that starts with the phrase "I want you to . . ." and finish the sentence. It can be silly, serious, or somewhere in between. It's just practice. Here are some examples:

"I want you to teach me how to make that cake you brought to the party."

"I want you to know I had a hilarious dream starring you last night."

"I want you to meet me for brunch this weekend, please!"

And no, hints don't work. If you think you're asking for what you want by dropping hints and then getting annoyed your partner isn't picking up on them, you're being a jerk. People aren't mind readers, and letting resentment fester because someone isn't noticing your ambiguous and subtle signals sets everyone up for failure. Be clear.

WHAT ABOUT WHEN YOU HAVE NO FUCKING CLUE?

We all know that feeling of searching for an answer and coming up blank. Sometimes it's because the answer is something we didn't even know existed. In other cases, the thing we want feels so shameful or embarrassing, we bury it even from ourselves. Most often it's because we genuinely just don't know what we want. The answer to all these conundrums is education, conversation, and, especially, *experimentation*.

Experimentation can look pretty simple:

> "Can you pull my hair?"

But it can also look fairly complicated:

> "Can you pull my hair while you fuck me in this sling and orgasm right as the beat drops in this song?"

If you don't know what you want:

1   Take a breath and think into the space posed by the question. Don't rush this part. Give yourself time to think it over.

2   If you know the answer after taking some time, then answer. If you don't, think of what you might like that wasn't even part of the question.

3   If you're still coming up blank, ask your partner to try an option, with the caveat that if you don't like it, you'll say so. Sometimes we don't know what we want because we don't know what the result will be. Cocreate a result and then decide if you like it or not.

4   When in doubt, back up to the last thing you remember liking. Or . . .

5   Cuddle and reassess. Cuddling can be your neutral zone. It's intimate and sensual, and it feels good. If you get overwhelmed or anxious, go to the cuddle zone and ground yourself.

6   Above all, stop muscling through. Sex is not something you should have to grin and bear. The bedroom could do with a little more conscious touch and communication. If something isn't working for you, stop and adjust. You won't ruin the moment. If you do ruin the moment, *the moment was supposed to be ruined*.

LEND A HAND

Sometimes your partner won't be as forthcoming as you'd like. If you get mixed signals or are flying blind, take a minute to make sure you're all on the same page. Here are a few ways to create short, sweet check-ins during the do:

Ask either/or and yes/no questions. Pussy got your tongue? Some folks can get a little preverbal when they get turned on, making it hard to articulate what they want. Either/or questions can help. "Faster or slower?" "Stay here or move up a bit?" "More lube?" Anything someone can answer clearly with a shake/nod of the head or a simple one-word response is a good question.

PRO TIP

Here's a question I want you to eradicate from your lexicon: "Is this okay?" It's the sexy-time equivalent of "How are you? Fine, thanks." Any answer to this question gives you zero constructive information. Instead, try "Do you like this?" That question is easily answered with a yes or no. With either answer, the next question can be "What would make it better?"

Play the number game. If you or your partner are truly in the dark about what feels good, try playing a game. Stimulate your partner in a way you think they'll enjoy, like, say, kissing their neck. You can ask, "On a scale of one to ten, how is this?" All the other person has to do is come up with a number. Let's say it's a four. Then, you can ask, "What would make it a six?" or "Would you like me to try for a five?"

When in doubt, dial it back. If your partner is frozen or too quiet to read or is making an ambiguous face or sound, take the energy down a notch and try to get a clearer understanding by asking a simple question. If you don't get anything from that, stop, get eye contact, and ask again. You're not going to lose the moment by pausing. You can always ramp the energy back up if that's what y'all want.

> I was once cranky as hell at a BDSM party. I didn't know what I wanted or how to improve my mood. A friend offered to give me a play piercing. While I don't find pain or blood erotic, I trusted my friends when they insisted the endorphin rush was a great mood-lifter. So I figured it was worth a try. The end result was . . . decidedly not my thing. But I'm glad I explored the option, and crossed it off my list for future explorations.

The Four Principles of Speaking Up*

1   **If you're a yes, say yes:**
    This reduces ambiguity and gets you what you want.

2   **If you're a no, say no:**
    You don't have to explain your no or couch it with apologies.

3   **If you're a maybe, say no:**
    "Maybe" keeps people hanging. Say "no" to give yourself time to figure out what you actually want, because . . .

4   **You are always free to change your mind:**
    A yes might become a no because you don't like the way it feels. A no might become a yes when you start to relax with your partner. A maybe might become either when you have more information. Change your mind as often as you want.

(*borrowed with permission from CuddleParty.com)

Changing Your Mind

Our culture has a weird connection to tenacity. Maybe it comes from when we're kids, driving our parents nuts with our impulsivity:

> "I choose Anger Man!
> No, Speedy Girl. Wait, no!
> I want Roarmonger!"

> "JUST CHOOSE!"

We're taught to make up our mind and stick with it. True, stick-to-itiveness can be a positive trait in many things. One exception? Sex. Changing your mind in sex is a *great* thing. It can open up new possibilities, get you out of situations you don't want to be in, and get you into more situations you *do* want to be in. Sex is made up of a *ton* of components. Changes or realizations to any one aspect of it can influence an overall shift in whether you want to be doing what you're doing at all.

You likely know this feeling already.

Have you ever lusted after someone from a distance, but the minute they opened their mouth is was like « GAME OVER » ? Have you had hella chemistry with someone but when you realized you both had completely different kissing styles, it was like, "What even *is* this, then?" Have you ever had the mood killed by bad breath or political disagreement or the speed at which things were moving?

This is what changing your mind is for, folks!

Consent is instantly revocable, which means *you are under NO obligation to keep going*. Even if you were going to sleep over. Even if you thought you wanted it. Even if you're lonely. Even if they bought you an expensive dinner. Even if they paid you for it. You are under no obligation to do anything with your body you don't want to do. Full stop.

Some people tend to go with the flow to a fault, and learn to disassociate or placate their concerns. So instead of saying "Hey, can we stop? I'm not really feeling this anymore," they grin and bear it or just tell themselves whatever happens will be easier than having an awkward conversation.

The problem is, when we don't speak up right away, it almost always turns into a bigger issue. So, practice saying what's on your mind right away. Like needing to pee at the movies, the longer you hold on to it, the worse it'll feel.

Same with speaking up during sex. Leg getting a cramp? Say so! Realize your heart is hurting because you're thinking of your ex? Take a breather! Body odor turning you off? Suggest showering together! Suddenly realizing you don't want to be there? Thank them and leave! Do it fast, do it right away, and enjoy instant satisfaction. If you're polite and clear, most kind people are happy to accommodate you changing your mind.

Disappointing people sucks, no doubt. But disappointing yourself by compromising your needs can hurt more. Do yourself a favor and give yourself the permission to change your mind.

PRO TIP

There's a big difference between pushing your boundaries and getting clear messages to get the fuck out of somewhere. It's important to listen to your animal instincts when exploring new things and people. If you're having a hard time figuring out one from the other, I suggest reading Gavin de Becker's *The Gift of Fear*, which is about learning to tune in to that voice in your head that tells you when something is just not okay.

Making Upgrades

Generally happy with the way things are going but need to make a small shift? Use the Appreciation Sandwich, a technique I learned from relationship educator LiYana Silver.

The Appreciation Sandwich has three parts:

1   Acknowledgment

2   Upgrade

3   Appreciation

Here's how it works: You acknowledge what's working, then request a shift or upgrade, then appreciate them for making the change. You can use it anytime, from a first date all the way to long-term relationships. Heck, you can even use it at work.

Let's see it in action (in decidedly *not* workplace environments):

> "I loved fucking you last night. Next time can we try integrating the toy I just bought? I'm excited to see what we can come up with together."

The Appreciation Sandwich works just as well in the middle of sex:

> "This feels wonderful. Would you mind eating me out a little longer? I love the way you're touching me."

> "I love the way you're pulling my hair. Can you please pull harder? Oh, yes!"

DIRTY TALK INTEGRATION

Dirty talk is perfectly suited for double duty: getting permission/clarity/ consent *and* amplifying the sexy vibes. Hopefully you've already gotten some information from your partner about the words they like to use. Remember, not everyone likes the same words used in bed. So get clear ahead of time whether calling someone "dirty slut" or "sweet boy" will be hot or not.

For folks who enjoy role-play, power exchange, or consensual nonconsent, safe words are *gold*. They were invented so people could play with saying no without actually meaning it. If you want to play this way, establish a safe word before things get too heated, otherwise it's fine to let "no" or "stop" keep their usual meanings.

To integrate negotiation into hot dialogue, try these tips:

Offer positive affirmation. General affirmation is nice, but specifics can take it up a notch. Do you like the way they're nibbling your ear? Say so! Or, at least, moan so. Consider this the "positive reinforcement" part of training your lover. Same thing if you're topping. Does he look sexy? Tell him! Are you happy she accepted your invitation for a date? That's a sweet thing to whisper into her ear when you're kissing her neck.

Note the power dynamic. Anyone can check in and make requests, but the sexy dynamic may alter the words you use. For instance:

> "All right baby, I'm going to need you to slow down. I want to make sure you're enjoying every inch of this."

> "Can we please slow down, Sir? I'm getting too excited!"

. . . are two ways of asking for the same thing.

Yummy noises are your friend. Worried about being articulate? Worry no more. It's a scientifically proven fact that sexy sounds are sexy to hear. Moans, grunts, purrs, and sighs serve the delightfully double duty of sounding hot and letting your partner know they're doing things right.

PRO TIP

Sexy sounds aren't just sexy for your partner to hear, they help keep the sexy going for you, too. Next time you're jacking off, try making all the porno sounds you can. (Preferably if the kids/roommates are out.) It might feel a little silly, but, hey, jacking off can feel a little silly. Stay authentic, just amplified. This goes extra for dudes, who often have a hard time making yummy noises, despite how much their partners *love* hearing them. The bonus is making noise means you're breathing, which is pretty fucking important to help your nerves send pleasure through your body.

Ask questions. "Do you like the way my hand feels on your throat?" "Are you ready for the vibrator?"

Tone of voice is key. Dirty talk can be roared or whispered. It all depends on the dynamic.

Integrate your power dynamic and pet names into the Appreciation Sandwich. Consider something like, "Oh sweet thing, you're doing such a good job handling these spankings. I want you to count out the next five even louder. Good boi." Or the classic: "You fuck me so good. Harder! Yes! Yes!"

Ta-daa! Communication that is both helpful *and* hot! Go forth and spew helpful filth!

The Blanket Yes

A **blanket yes** is when you give consent for your partner to do whatever during sex. It's best used when you have a solid foundation of trust with your partner and feel empowered about speaking up in the moment. Many long-term partners give each other a blanket yes after they've laid all of the groundwork and they don't have anything new to negotiate. It doesn't negate any prior negotiations or safe words, but gives your partner permission to try things within an established framework. It's like driving straight ahead until your GPS tells you to make a turn. If no one is saying anything, nothing is wrong. When someone speaks up, the blanket yes is over until reinstated.

The blanket yes is usually most helpful when you're tired of saying yes over and over and just want to go with it. For me, it's my "Shut up and kiss me" moment. That is, when I notice I'm annoyed they keep asking my permission to do things that I definitely want done. It's a clear indicator light I feel confident in my ability to articulate my desires and confident in my partner's ability to honor my requests. Do *not* use a blanket yes when you're too nervous to have a conversation, worried the person will be annoyed or mad if you don't, or tired of the sex and just want it to be over.

PRO TIP

You are *never* required to accept a blanket yes. Consent goes both ways. Tops have just as much right to feel safe and certain before proceeding with any sex acts.

Are We There Yet?
Ego and Orgasm

So, how do you know when sex is actually over and the aftercare can begin? Well, common courtesy dictates it's a decision made together. For some, that might mean everyone has an orgasm. For others, it may be whatever makes everyone feel "complete." It's generally a good idea to check in when you feel like things may be coming to a close. This is particularly useful if you may be out of commission after a certain point (such as post-orgasm or when you reach a certain state of exhaustion). Try to come up with a win-win for how to close out the sex sesh. This may mean you bring out the vibrator, steer the energy toward a more grounded place, or switch gears so you can arrive at the same point together. If orgasm isn't on the table for you, it's all right to give your partner a heads-up and let them know what you might want instead.

Many folks stake their pride in how well they can get a partner off. While it's great to be conscientious about a partner's pleasure, be careful not to make *their* orgasm about *you*. Not everyone comes during sex, or comes every time. Check in and ask what your partner would like, but take care not to pressure them to perform pleasure just to make you feel better about yourself.

Post-Coital Communication

Sometimes you and your partner will be totally compatible during the do, but your post-game differs. There's nothing wrong with that, but it helps to know what you like and be able to communicate it. Are you a cuddler? Do you hate feeling sticky or icky after sex? Do you want to shower right after? Or do you love to luxuriate in the oh-so-sexy funk? Will you fall asleep immediately? Will you want to run laps? Will you want to jack off one more time and then make snacks? The answers to these questions can vary depending on your connection to your partner, your mood, or just the time of day.

Remember, your partner doesn't cease to exist after you've had sex with them. Let them know your post-sex preferences and ask for theirs in return. If you can find common ground, all the better.

Aftercare

Aftercare is what folks need to feel safe, content, and complete after sex. Your job is to make your partner feel just as cared for after the sex as during. Eye contact and physical contact are usually a good idea. Cuddling is standard issue for most folks, but if you need alone time, a shower, or to do yoga or whatever, that's fine, too. Be communicative!

Pillow talk is a great time to discuss the sex you just had, especially if you hope to do it again. You can use this time to:

Clear up confusion. Not sure why your partner asked for something? Wondering why they made a certain sound? Feeling like you picked up on something that contradicted what you talked about before sex? Pillow talk is a great time to sort it out.

Discuss your favorite parts. This can reinforce good choices and make it easier to remember what you both liked for next time.

Add things to try next time. (If there is a next time.)

Sex can be an intense experience. It's normal to feel emotional, vulnerable, or activated afterward. Tears, laughter, chattiness, quietness, alertness, sleepiness are all natural aftereffects of sex. One-night stands can be the hardest for aftercare because there can be a bit of that "you saw my O-face and now I'm embarrassed" vibe. The best way to handle the awkward is to acknowledge it, and just relax. A big part of sexual self-confidence comes from role-modeling that nothing's wrong even when there are emotions involved.

During sex with a newish lover, I wanted him to slap my face, but I didn't feel like there was a perfect time for it, so I let it go. Then, later during our after-sex cuddle, I mentioned how much I had wanted him to do it. He told me he had assumed face-slapping was a hard no for me. My request allowed us to clear up some confusion *and* add new things to the menu for next time.

The Morning After

Within these pages, there's no such thing as a walk of shame, only a stride of pride. You had a good time with someone, maybe tried some new things, and learned some stuff. Good on ya. Regardless of whether or not you want to see your sex buddy again, current standard protocol for the morning after is a thank-you text the next day. If you had a good time, say so. You can add another simple compliment if you want:

"Thanks for a great night. I slept sooo well afterward!"

"That was yummy. I loved the last position. ;)"

"Thanks! You're awesome!"

Whatever you decide, make sure you're being both honest and direct. If you want to see them again, say so:

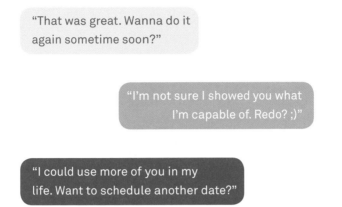

"That was great. Wanna do it again sometime soon?"

"I'm not sure I showed you what I'm capable of. Redo? ;)"

"I could use more of you in my life. Want to schedule another date?"

If they say yes, I recommend scheduling a date right then. Aim for two to three weeks later. Too soon and you may risk imprinting, too late and you might end up in the no-man's-land of complex schedules. If you're not interested in a redo, leave it at thanks. If you need to dole out some gentle rejection, revisit page 80.

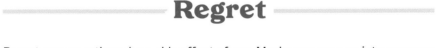

Regret

Regret can sometimes be a side effect of sex. Maybe you were so into someone you relaxed your own rules; or maybe you felt so lonely you lowered your standards; or maybe in the harsh light of day, you just felt like you made a mistake. Whatever the case may be, start by acknowledging and validating your feelings. Regret happens, and no good will come from pretending you aren't feeling it. Next:

→ **Investigate the cause.** Did you lie or cheat? Did you pressure yourself or your partner? Did you get drunker than intended? Did you not feel appreciated by your partner? Did you break a promise to yourself? Do you feel judged by your peers or your God? Put a name to whatever the reason.

→ **Make amends if necessary.** If you did something to or with another person you regret, you need to figure out how to make it right. If you violated their consent, acknowledge this and possibly embark on restorative justice (see page 155). If the only one you hurt is yourself, acknowledge that, too.

→ **Forgive yourself.** If you didn't hurt anyone but yourself, forgive yourself.

→ **Commit to change.** Try to pinpoint the behavior that caused you to make a choice you regret, and decide on future actions to minimize the likelihood of doing it again.

The best way to minimize regrettable experiences before they happen is to honor everyone's boundaries, including your own. Stay sober. Inebriation is the quickest way to make choices you'll regret later. Don't let loneliness, depression, or feeling like a failure make you relax your boundaries. It's almost always better to go home alone than it is to wake up next to someone you really didn't like in the first place. If you're not crystal clear on your partner's boundaries, *ask*. If you're picking up on a weird vibe or can't remember what you discussed about their wants and dislikes, get clarity before pushing ahead. Above all, talk about it. Sneaking out in the wee hours of the morning and then ignoring every text they send afterward doesn't lessen feelings of regret. Rather, it usually compounds any shitty feelings either of you may have. If you feel like something is off, address it as soon as possible. Give one another the opportunity to clear up miscommunications or hurt feelings right away.

If you know you're having casual sex to avoid other issues in your life, it might be time for you to consider taking a sex break for a little while to reacclimatize your relationship to your body. (See page 251 for information about conscious celibacy.)

Meanwhile, if you feel regret because of external forces, like your peer group or church, consider who you're letting dictate what you do with your body. If your regret would dissipate if you had a group of friends to brag to over brunch, is it really the sex you regret, or your current friends' judgment? If you feel extra-awesome while you're having the sex, but feel extra-guilty in church the next morning, it's probably not the sex that's the problem.

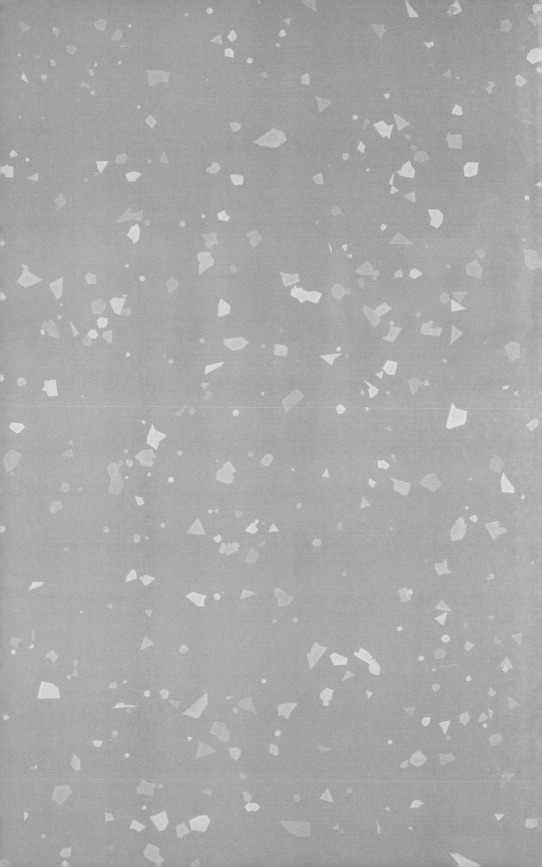

Booze, Weed, and Other Drugs

There's a reason why so much of the conversation about hookups revolves around alcohol and drug use. Many folks use these things to lower their inhibitions and connect with people. Many folks also just like the feeling of getting a little buzzed. There's nothing wrong with any of this on the surface, but alcohol becomes a problem when people need so much of it they lose sense of their boundaries and ability to self-assess.

Alcohol

Just like gender and sexual orientation, inebriation isn't a binary. There are many gradations of drunkenness between stone-cold sober and passed out on the bathroom floor. The key is to be able to identify where you are on the scale at any moment and make appropriate choices. Just as a savvy drinker knows when to hand over their car keys, they also know when to go to bed alone. Here's a simple scale to show you the downward slope of drunkenness:

Aaahh. The glass of wine after a hard day at work. The beer with the game. This amount of alcohol doesn't feel like much to most people, but it has an effect. Depending on your body mass and experience, this amount can make you feel a little relaxed, warm, or sleepy.

Buzzed. The buzz is what most casual drinkers are looking for when they drink. It's a feel-good, light, giggly feeling. You are slightly impaired (so ixnay on the driving) but you're able to carry on conversations and maintain general executive function, like mobility, linear thinking, and eye contact.

WHOO! Do you want table dancing? Because this is how you get table dancing. Just one click before blackouts exist the wide-open plains of WHOO! drunk. This is the most common form found at college parties, late night at the club, or in the dry-out tank at your local jail. When people are WHOO! drunk, they can't drive, can't operate machinery, and can't make important choices, like whether to have another or not. When you're WHOO! drunk, you may make bad choices, and you'll likely remember (and regret) them the next day.

Blacked Out. Blackouts are the most dangerous neighborhood in Drunk-landia. You're in a blackout when you are seemingly alert and responsive, but your long-term memory is on the fritz. This means folks around you may not even know you're drunk, because you're talking and moving like you would normally. But you won't remember any of it. You won't remember if you gave consent to go home with someone. You won't remember if *they* gave you *their* consent. The person you went home with may not even know you were in a blackout, and thus *unable* to consent. You can black out for moments, hours, or even a whole night, and the next day you won't remember any of it. Do I need to tell you this is bad news?

> I've blacked out twice and both times were *terrifying*. Once, I woke up naked in my ex-boyfriend's bed, not knowing how I got there or where my clothes were. To this day, I don't know what happened that night.

Passed Out. This is when your body puts a fork in you, because you are done. You may be difficult to rouse or in danger of alcohol poisoning.

Anywhere on the scale could be a danger zone depending on your tolerance and advocacy skills. Anything beyond a buzz can be really bad news. You may make choices you regret, get into situations you can't get yourself out of, and lose track of the consequences of your actions. Do everyone a favor, and stick with "Aaahh" or lightly "Buzzed" if you're planning on drinking at all.

Some folks think it's impossible to use alcohol responsibly. I am not one of those people. I think many people can self-medicate with alcohol with few complications. Here are my thoughts on how to mix sex and alcohol:

Have a plan. Celebrating a promotion? Just got dumped and need to forget your life for a while? If you're going out to drink, know why you're doing it.

Have friends. Getting drunk while out and alone is a recipe for trouble. It's also less fun. If you want to party with booze, bring some trusted friends. A designated driver (both literally and figuratively) is always a good idea. Don't let any of your friends leave with someone you don't know. Don't leave any of your buddies behind. Get some #SquadGoals up in your drinking game. If you're not sure you can trust your friends, consider enlisting support from the bartender. Decent bartenders will be happy to support you by giving you water between cocktails or cutting you off before they might otherwise.

Don't be a hero. Contrary to what Westerns say, drinking is not a competition. There is no such thing as "winning" a drinking match. Remember, alcohol is poison. If you win, you lose.

Have a limit. Decide where on the scale of "Aaahh" to "Passed Out" you want to get, knowing it's never a good idea to venture beyond "WHOO!" It stops being fun after that point anyway. The challenge is knowing how to hit your target. This takes practice. When you first start exploring alcohol, drink slowly and methodically. It's much more fun to drink good alcohol with good friends than bargain-basement hooch at crazy parties anyway.

Slow your roll. Drinking fast is both expensive and dangerous. You can slow down by getting a single cocktail in a double glass, eating a big meal before drinking, switching out to zero-proof beverages once you get to a nice cruising altitude, sticking to low-proof beverages, using cash at the bar (instead of opening a tab), and my personal favorite: upgrading your cocktail experience with sippable bevvies, like a nice scotch, bitter cocktails (made with Cynar or Campari), or strong red wines. Bonus: Drinks such as these make you look way classier than the folks slamming Long Island iced teas.

Now that I'm familiar with my limits, I'll sometimes order one fancy cocktail to start off the night, then follow up with one glass of wine. After that, I order seltzer with lime (usually free) or mixed with juice until my crew is ready to pack it in.

PROBLEM DRINKING

For some, alcoholism is a purely biological disease. Others abuse alcohol because they're avoiding real problems in their lives and want to numb the pain. This method might work temporarily, but *only* temporarily. As soon as they sober up, there are those glaring problems again, right where they left them. Regardless of where your alcohol problem comes from, the best thing to do is reach out and get help. This can look like twelve-step programs, other kinds of support groups (most LGBTQ+ centers have substance abuse programs that are gender and sexual-identity affirming), or one-on-one therapy.

Roughly 25 percent of queer and trans folks abuse alcohol, as contrasted with 5 to 10 percent of straight people.[1] The fact is, the more troubles a population has, and the more isolated from community, prosperity, and health care they are, the more likely that population is to abuse substances. So reach out and get help, if not just for you, for your community.

Your immediate culture also has a big effect on how you engage with substances. Some folks find it hard to socialize after they cut drinking from their lives. The good news is there are lots of people who are looking to date and socialize with other sober people. So while you may feel isolated from your immediate circle, you will be delighted to find a whole new world of cool folks to kick it with. Plus, you may become the role-model that others in your community need when examining their alcohol intake.

When I was in my twenties, it was hard to find people to hang out with who weren't drug and alcohol users. Now? I'd say at least half of my friends and lovers don't imbibe at all. The other half is folks who'll have a glass of wine with dinner but that's pretty much it. Sexy sober people are out there, and they're usually better conversationalists and sex partners than the sloshed folks at bars. Go out and make some (sober) friends!

IT'S NOT ME, IT'S YOU

If your potential paramour is inebriated, exercise extreme caution. The best thing to do is help everyone get home safe. Often that's by enlisting one of their sober friends to help, or by being that sober friend yourself. But remember, inebriation isn't an excuse for bad behavior. If a drunk person is violating your boundaries, tell them to stop or get help from your friends or venue staff. If your date got too drunk to truly consent to sexy shenanigans, take a rain check. Sure, they may be coming on strong and insisting they're a yes, but a drunken yes just isn't the same thing as a sober yes. There's always the next morning. If you're both drunk enough to be impaired, you're *both* technically unable to consent. You being equally smashed doesn't absolve either of your responsibility for doing things you shouldn't have.

Hangover Blues

Okay, sure, I can tell you all this stuff, but that doesn't mean you're going to listen to me. So what do you do when you both wake up with pounding heads and blurry memories of the prior night? First, check in. Don't you dare coyote ugly this one. Stick around, talk it out, and follow the same considerate aftercare process (see page 133) as you should with all sexual encounters. Share what's going on for you. Do you remember what happened? What are you feeling? Ask how they are, and be open to all the answers they may share. Often the difference between a mutually laughable hookup and an event that leaves someone feeling violated is how they're treated *after* the fact. Treat them with dignity and humanity, even if you feel ashamed yourself. Be real about what's up.

Next, start a conversation about safer sex. If you failed to take precautions, yeah, it's too late for prevention, but there are still potential harm-reduction actions to take. Is pregnancy a possibility? Take Plan B or another morning-after pill (see page 201). Do you have an undisclosed STI? Now's the time to disclose. There are plenty of ways to treat many STIs after exposure, even HIV (see page 189). The only way you can treat them, though, is if you know what's going on. Share your sexual health info so your partner can make informed decisions about what to do next, and then get tested as soon as you can.

If you actually dig each other, say so. Make sure they know you're happy you hooked up. Even if you're feeling shame about your inebriation, that doesn't mean you have to feel shame about the sexy-times. Let them know you're down for more sober fun in the future. Reread this chapter from the start, and next time, give yourself the opportunity to fully consent by staying more sober. I believe in you.

Weed

It's harder to get as blotto with weed as it is with alcohol, but that doesn't mean it can't happen. Getting too high can make you lethargic to the point of passing out, feeling weak and confused, and having difficulty articulating your needs. Just like with alcohol, it's important to know your limits and to know where your good space is so you don't put yourself in a dangerous situation.

If you live in a place with legalized weed, go to a reputable dispensary to gear up. It's *very* easy to ingest too much in the form of homemade edibles, so if you're still getting to know your body and the right dose for you, go slow and wait a solid hour after eating to monitor the effects. Most of the horror stories about weed come from people eating more than they could handle and being miserably high for way too long. Also, if you're already drunk, or even just buzzed, adding weed to the equation can be a roundhouse kick to the noggin. Stoner pros call this "the spins" because it feels like you just disembarked the Teacups ride at Disneyland. It can incapacitate you and make you feel like utter garbage. I wish someone had warned me in college to stick to the "pass" in "puff puff pass" when using, so I could enjoy the night instead.

Don't be afraid to pass on weed entirely if it doesn't agree with you. Some folks feel paranoid, anxious, or just weird when they get high. If that's you, it's okay to say so. Regardless of the drug, the best way to avoid imbibing (too much or at all) is to not hang out with people who don't respect your boundaries. Just like with sex, you shouldn't have to come up with an excuse for your no. If your friends don't respect it, they're likely not to respect it in other contexts.

Party Drugs, Psychedelics, and Pharmaceuticals

No matter the drug, someone's tried to fuck while high on it. So let's dive into the wild world of tripping tits. First, here's the dope: Taking drugs is risky. I don't mean in a *Reefer Madness* kind of way. I mean lots of drugs these days aren't what you think they are. Party drugs such as MDMA and cocaine are processed, meaning they can be cut with other substances to stretch the product and improve the profit margin for sellers. Capitalism, yo.

Often these additives are annoying but not deadly—things such as aspirin or vitamin C. However, there's been a rise in additives that are *supremely* dangerous, most notably party drugs cut with fentanyl. Fentanyl is an opioid used as a painkiller in hospitals. It's a hundred times more powerful than morphine, stronger than heroin, cheaper than cocaine, and horribly unsafe. Illicitly manufactured fentanyl can cause respiratory issues and cardiac arrest. The drug is responsible for *thousands* of deaths in Canada and the United States. Some dealers cut their drugs with it to create a similar euphoria without having to shell out for the real deal. It's like adding bleach to your soda to make it last longer.

So yeah, bad news bears.

If you still want to enjoy party drugs, use a drug testing kit. Kits are affordable, good for multiple uses, and easily ordered online. If you're going to drop $$$ for drugs, you can add a small fee to make sure you don't literally kill yourself and your friends, right? Decent drug dealers will also test their drugs before selling, so it's worth it to find someone you can trust to sell you real stuff instead of a pill mixed with livestock dewormer. (Yes, really.)

Once you've got a substance you know is relatively safe, and *only* when you do, the usual rules apply: know your limits, start slow, and do it with friends you trust.

A couple more considerations for the intrepid psychonauts among us:

Don't be spontaneous. Plan for a drug trip; don't just take what someone gives you at the club. There's little worse than tripping balls in a place you don't want to be with no way of leaving. If you want to go on a drug journey, do it with trusted friends in a safe, comfortable environment. It's more fun that way anyway.

Know your intention. Psychedelics and party drugs can be sources of profundity, illumination, and intimacy. Or they can be hours of anxiety and bad vibes. The best way to steer your experience in a good direction is having a clear intention. For example, a group of friends may choose to do MDMA (aka Molly/Ecstasy) together to have a shared sexy/cuddly high. You may go on a daytime hike with shrooms to vibe off of nature. You might decide to do LSD to give yourself perspective on your consciousness. If you dose with a clear intention, you can help steer yourself toward these experiences; and in my opinion, you're using them the way they're intended.

Maintain your boundaries. Yeah, I know psychedelics and boundaries may sound like a contradiction, but drugs aren't an excuse for violating anyone's boundaries. Some drugs, particularly MDMA/MDA, are known for making touch feel *really* damn good. This can be fun when you're with intimate partners or friends, but it can be overwhelming with folks you're not interested in smooching. Likewise, some drugs, like GHB, can mimic the effects of alcohol, making you just as susceptible to overdoing it.

Don't mix substances. Combining depressants (such as GHB and alcohol) can be life-threatening. Particularly if you're a newbie. As my mama used to say, "Stick with the lady who brought ya."

Don't be afraid to call for help. While it's hard to OD on psychedelics, dangerous events, like dehydration, aren't uncommon. In the United States, police are often first responders to 911 calls, even if what you need is medical treatment. Everyone has a different relationship to law enforcement, particularly when illegal activity is happening. I don't necessarily advocate calling the cops, but if your friend needs medical care, it's your job to get them some. This may mean calling for a rideshare or a cab to get to the hospital, calling a sober friend for help, or if the situation is dire, biting the bullet and calling 911 and asking for paramedics.

For straightforward information about all drugs, check out Erowid.com.

ANTIDEPRESSANTS AND SSRIS

Antidepressants have a reputation for making sexual pleasure harder to come by. They can kill your libido and make it difficult to orgasm and get hard/wet. But they may also keep you functional and alive. So, hey, it's a trade-off.

If you are being treated for anxiety and/or depression, it may be worth your time to experiment with different dosages and drugs to see what gets you the right mix to feel as good as you can. There is a huge variety out on the market now, so talk to your doctor about your options. You may find one that gives you the cruising altitude you need to be both functional and sexual.

BONER PILLS

What penis-owner hasn't at some point at least *thought* about Viagra/Cialis? These drugs, once limited to the realm of sci-fi pornos, are now in medicine cabinets and slut-kits the world over. However, there's a reason why they're still prescription-only. Viagra was invented as a heart medication. Researchers found that improving vascularity had a curious side effect, and thus the boner pill was born.

While a healthy person can take the occasional boner pill without fear of big side effects, there are still risks, particularly if you have an undiagnosed heart condition, hypertension, or blood pressure problems. Before taking a boner pill, talk to your doctor to minimize any potential health risks.

SPEED

Methamphetamines are a class of drug commonly known as speed. Study aids/ADD drugs, like Adderall, and street drugs, like crystal (aka Tina), are methamphetamines. Some folks enjoy mixing meth and sex because it lowers their inhibitions. The problems are (1) you have inhibitions for a reason and (2) meth tends to lower them all the way to hell. If you feel as if you need meth to enjoy sex, interrogate your inhibitions and figure out where you can work to enjoy sex without having to ignore the realities of your life. If you feel inadequate or have sexual shame, meth can be the thing you think you need to ignore that awful reality for a little while. Of course, that shame doesn't go anywhere, and the next day you may feel extra awful, and in the meantime you may have exposed yourself to some dangerous situations or to a brutal addiction. Spare yourself.

Erections and Orgasms Under the Influence

If erections are important to you or your sex partner, many drugs can get in the way of a good time. Whiskey dick is real, but it's not only alcohol's fault. Stimulants (like cocaine), antidepressants (like Wellbutrin), depressants (like benzos), anesthetics (like ketamine), and even nicotine can make erections difficult to achieve and maintain.

Some drugs may not interfere with an erection, but they challenge the body in other ways, like by increasing heart rate and overheating, or by making a person distractible and dissociated.

Many drugs can make orgasm much harder for vulva-owners, too. Sexual pleasure is about blood flow and hormones, after all, so anything that restricts vascularity (like nicotine) or dopamine reuptake (like antidepressants) can make orgasms a whole lot harder to come by.

Disinhibition

Many drugs have "prosexual" effects, which means they facilitate or amplify sexual behavior. The most common prosexual effect is disinhibition—aka letting your guard down and relaxing. What we often feel as sexual excitement is just disinhibition at work. You stop hyper-analyzing yourself or feeling like a weirdo. You chat up a cute person you'd never have the nerve to talk to sober, and so on. Disinhibition can make you feel braver and sexier. In this way disinhibition can be a great thing, especially if you're on the anxious or depressed side of things.

Disinhibition can be dangerous, however, when it lowers not only your inhibitions but also your standards. When you lose your inhibitions, you may also lose your insistence on using a condom, your ability to assert yourself, and your willingness to leave a fucked-up situation. This is why sexual assault cases that involve drugs and alcohol get so messy so quickly—many folks wonder why they made certain foolish choices in the first place when they were smashed.

Simply put: Drugs of all kinds can make you more likely to engage in risky sexual behavior, full stop. Now, I can give you tips to try to keep your head on straight when you're fucked up, but the fact is, when you're fucked up, you're not likely to listen to *anyone's* good advice, let alone mine.

The one piece of advice I can give you has to be taken while you're sober: Develop a life where you feel sexy and brave even when you're sober. That's far easier said than done, of course, but it's worth trying. If you're in the closet or ashamed of your desires, if you're lying to yourself about who you are and what you want, if you don't respect yourself or the people around you—you're more likely to get blotto and make risky sexual choices. So, start your path of self-love and you'll find the results ripple well into your sex life.

Spectrums of Harm

Lapses in communication and collaboration are where harm happens.

When we go on autopilot and forget to check in with our partner . . .

When we intentionally *or* accidentally violate a boundary . . .

When we forget to ask for clarity and step into an awkward situation . . .

When we ignore the needs or desires of a partner because we are too invested in our own good time . . .

. . . we can do harm.

Like most everything, harm exists on a spectrum. On one end, everything's A-OK and no one is harmed. On the opposite end is intentional, cruel, and violent harm. Most choices we make fall somewhere in between the two. Because of the complexity of sex, and the intersecting natures of hearts, egos, bodies, trauma, and identity, it can be painfully easy to cause harm.

Keep in mind that you don't get to decide how harmed someone else feels. You can't control other people's feelings, you can only control the choices you make when faced with them. Also, understand that harm is deeply contextual. If a dear friend accidentally misgenders me, odds are good I'll get over it quickly. If, however, someone elbow-checks me in the grocery store and says, "Excuse me, SIR!" (yes, that happened), I might feel a bit more harmed. Same offense, different context. Again, only you get to decide how hurt you feel by the incident.

If you've been harmed, there are varying ways of dealing with it. Some methods better suit the situation than others. Be cautious about putting anyone on blast right away. If you think the person who hurt you is a menace who needs to be called out publicly, that's your decision to make. However, if you just need to be seen and validated, there are better ways to do it than taking to social media. Getting a bunch of strangers worked up online may feel righteous, but it won't repair harm, it won't heal your wounds, and it often creates far more pain for everyone involved, especially the harmed parties. Instead, consider enlisting support from your community, requesting a restorative justice or accountability process (see page 155), and finding ways to get the witnessing you need. Once you've done that, what's the best way to tell an otherwise decent person they hurt you, possibly by accident?

Acknowledge your feelings. If it feels like a big deal, it doesn't do any good to convince yourself it's not. You're allowed to feel violated, betrayed, angry, or whatever. Your feelings are valid.

Investigate what went wrong from your perspective. Did you want to speak up but couldn't? Did you speak up but they didn't hear you? Did you think everything was fine but realized after the fact that it wasn't? Get clear on when and how the misstep happened.

When you're ready, have the conversation. If you think you need a friend or mediator for support, by all means, get them involved. You can write down your experience, too, and it can be good to follow up your conversation with everything in writing.

Try the Difficult Conversation Formula. Again, it's:

1   I have something to tell you.

2   Here's what I'm afraid will happen when I tell you . . .

3   Here's what I want to have happen . . .

4   Here's what I have to tell you . . .

This works because you're describing your emotional state to help the other person understand where you're coming from, and you're using "I" statements to make sure you're speaking from your own perspective.

Describe what happened from your perspective. It's important to keep using "I" statements here. At this point it's incredibly easy for everyone to get defensive, which doesn't do anyone much good. Avoid name-calling or stating opinions about the other person's experience. *Don't* assume you know what they were/are thinking or feeling. And, *remember to breathe*.

Allow them to share. You'll likely get lots of information here. The other person may reframe their perspective, take responsibility, avoid taking responsibility, and plenty of other things. Likely they won't react in the perfect way. It's hard to hear you hurt someone, even if it was unintentional. But acting poorly is different from being abusive or cruel. So if their reaction makes you feel unsafe, you have the right to end the conversation. (This is where a mediator can come in handy.)

Discuss future actions. If you're engaged in a positive dialogue, it's helpful, once everyone has shared, to consider future behaviors. This can look like deciding on new rules/boundaries, taking certain acts off the table for a while, or renegotiating the terms of your relationship. What's most important is you feel heard, seen, and respected by whatever you decide.

PRO TIP

You may have heard the phrase "impact over intent." This is meant to convey the idea that even though someone may have the best of intentions, if their words or actions hurt someone, they need to take responsibility for that hurt. However, this doesn't mean intent doesn't matter. There's a reason why our legal system delineates intent. It's the difference between negligence, manslaughter, and murder. In sex, knowing someone's intent is often the difference between whether you'll give someone the benefit of the doubt or never trust them again. While intent shouldn't overrule impact, it's okay to consider it when sorting out your feelings about complicated dynamics.

If roles are reversed, and an intimate partner tells you you've hurt them, here's a way to proceed:

1   **Stay calm and present.** Yes, it sucks to be told you hurt someone, but getting defensive won't take the pain away and will just make things worse. Breathe and listen.

2   **Thank them for speaking up and trusting you to hear them.** We live in a culture that doesn't want people to talk about their pain. Thanking them will go a long way toward rebuilding trust.

3   **Center the other person's experience.** Believe that their account of the situation happened as they say. The point isn't getting to the nitty-gritty facts of the matter; this isn't a courtroom. The priority is addressing the *emotional impact* of your choices. For instance, if they insist they used their safe word and you're convinced they didn't, it doesn't help to insist they're wrong. The point is, you didn't hear their safe word and you need to remedy that, regardless of the details.

4   **Apologize.** This can be hard, especially if you don't think you did anything wrong. Apologize anyway. A good way to do this is to apologize for the harm your actions or lack thereof had on them. You can say, "I'm sorry," or you can be more specific to show you understand

where they're coming from. "I'm sorry I touched you there/used that word/didn't ask before doing that" or whatever speaks to the specifics. (Check out *The 5 Languages of Apology* by Gary Chapman and Jennifer Thomas for a deep-dive into effective apologies.)

PRO TIP

You've likely heard many "non-apology apologies" in the media lately. The usual format is some variation of "I'm sorry you felt hurt." This kind of apology sucks because it takes zero accountability for *causing* the hurt. If I step on your foot, I shouldn't say, "I'm sorry your foot hurts." I should apologize *for hurting you*. Take responsibility for the impact of your actions or words. It will go a long way toward restoring trust.

5   **Commit to change.** An apology without improved behavior is meaningless. You need to demonstrate *growth* and *change*. Commit to actions that will demonstrate improvement. This may mean starting therapy, reading up on social justice, working with a coach, or other things your community and/or the harmed party suggest.

Recently, a guy hurt my feelings on our very first date. While what he did would normally be a deal breaker, I liked him so much and he apologized so well that I gave him a second chance. Then on our second date, he hurt my feelings again in a similar way. He showed me who he was from jump, but I wanted so badly to believe these were accidents that I ignored the clear signs the guy wasn't interested in changing his behavior and was ultimately no good for me. Had I given credence to his *actions*, not just his words, I might have saved myself from a brutal and protracted heartache.

If you're told you've done harm and/or violated someone's boundary, you don't get to decide if, how, or when you're forgiven. Forgiveness is ultimately up to the harmed party. You can apologize and ask forgiveness. You are not, however, *owed* forgiveness. Sometimes the person you hurt will forgive you right away, and sometimes it can take a while. And of course, it may never come at all. These are sometimes the consequences of harm.

Harm doesn't have to be a deal breaker, though. When everyone can feel honored and respected, even when airing grievances, it's much easier to heal the relationship and feel confident moving forward. One thing necessary to repair harm is showing up for the conversation. If the harm was egregious enough that you need to cut ties, that's fine. If, however, you believe the relationship is worth repairing, everyone involved needs to show up and talk it out. Nothing is healed by letting things fester. Address the harm and give everyone an opportunity to help heal it.

Restorative Justice

Restorative justice is a process developed by First Nations cultures in North America and the Maori in New Zealand to help solve conflict and heal harm within communities. Colonization forced a shift in focus from dealing with harm in community to judicial and carceral justice instead. As society becomes more aware of the flaws endemic to carceral justice, however, some communities and cultures are readapting to the more empathetic and effective community-minded restorative justice techniques.

Restorative justice is a complex and extraordinary technology that has powerful applications to sexual health and intimate relationships. It's well-worth investigating both on your own and within your chosen communities. There's not room in this book to do the topic justice, but I encourage you learn more about it, especially if you or someone you know needs to remedy harm in your community. See the page 270 for resources.

The Etiquette of Getting It

The protocols of pleasure. The courtesies of coitus. The suavity of sensuality. In this brave new world of eggplant emojis and "U up?" texts, it can be difficult to balance a filthy mind with a touch of class. But just because you're getting down and dirty doesn't mean you can't proceed with decorum. Let's explore the rules of play for sophisticated sluts.

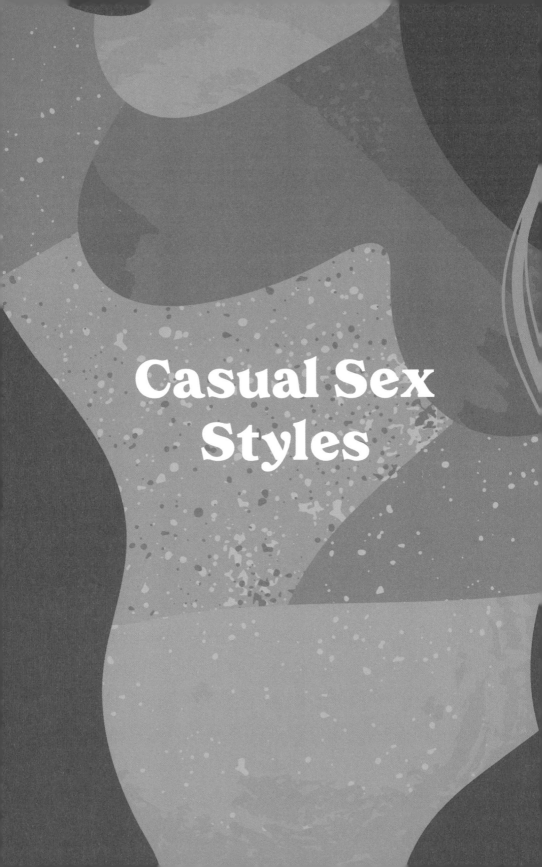

Casual Sex Styles

Many people think one-night stands when they hear "casual sex." It's the one-and-done style of hooking up. They tend to be many folks' default unless the sex or the connection is particularly special. However, lots of people like the idea of at least keeping the option open to see a sex partner again. In fact, there are plenty of casual relationship styles, one-night stands being only one of them.

Regardless of the form your casual arrangement takes, my advice rarely wavers: Keep it on the up-and-up by talking it out before the clothes start coming off. If you have a mitigating factor that *requires* the sex to be a one-night stand (like, say, you're moving away soon) say so. If you're resisting saying anything because you're afraid it will mean the other person won't want to sleep with you, that's a great sign you need to *say the fucking thing*. Lying to keep someone interested in you is a form of assault and supremely dickish. If you know you have a deal breaker, break the fucking deal and move on.

Regardless of whether or not you decide to see each other again, ghosting is bad form. Send the thank-you text, and if you see them at the grocery store next month, don't hide behind the kombucha. Treat your sex partners as people, even if you don't intend on seeing them naked again.

Friends with Benefits

"Friends with benefits" (FWB) is one of the more popular casual sex styles. It makes sense. You already enjoy spending time with that person, thus the "friends" part. The benefits come when you also enjoy each other . . . less clothed.

FWB arrangements can be temporary or ongoing. They can fit an immediate need or emerge from the natural relationship you already have. What can make FWB arrangements complicated is the fact that you do hang out other than naked-wise and have more involved social lives.

Here's how to handle a good FWB relationship:

Emphasis on the friends. There are few things crummier than having an FWB relationship go belly-up and take the friendship down with it. If things start getting wonky, prioritize your friendship to keep from losing an otherwise wonderful relationship. Don't ditch out on other plans because you're now banging. Enjoy your social life together, give each other high fives at the game, and remember you're *friends* first.

Don't let the awkward ruin it. Suddenly your bud knows what your O-face looks like. Go ahead and giggle about it. Then remember that sex with a cool person is an excellent thing to have in your life. Cherish the bond regardless of the silliness.

Let your other friends live in blissful ignorance. While you don't have to be in the closet about your sex life, you needn't feel obligated to regale your other friends with intimate details of the naughty-nurse role-play you did with their buddy last night, either. Sometimes it's nice to not have to contemplate all the sex other people are having. That said, don't get all super-spy about it either. Unless you have a compelling reason to keep it on the DL, it's a good idea to be transparent, so people don't think you're keeping secrets. If your FWB situation skews the overall dynamic of your friend group, take time to consider the whole group as a relationship and assess how you could improve the balance. Don't tank other good relationships to serve your sex life.

Check in periodically. Every relationship can benefit from an occasional State of the Union conversation. How are you feeling? How's the sex? How are the emotions? It's great to have check-in conversations even when everything seems to be going swimmingly, if only to make it easier to talk when things *aren't* perfect.

I Got No Strings!

No strings attached (NSA) arrangements are a specific subset of casual sex, emphasis on the *casual*. Most often, NSA means you and your partner act as sovereign entities, placing zero expectations on one another. You drop in, drop out, hook up when y'all wanna, and the rest of the time you don't stress about what they're up to. NSA works best when no one wants romance, and you're getting together for the sake of sex and nothing more. This is in contrast to the aforementioned FWB relationships, where you're hanging out as buds in between all the sexin'.

NSA is a viable choice for folks who aren't interested in a capital-R Relationship and prefer sex as the only way they want to hang out with each other. Like all kinds of sex, NSA relationships work best with some ground rules:

Protect your own body. Assume your partner is having sex with other people and choose your protocols accordingly. Remember, STIs follow the rule of transitivity: Anyone your partner shares skin contact/body fluids with, you are also in effect sharing skin contact/body fluids with. You can't control what your partner's partners are up to, so establish protocols that make you feel safe regardless.

Respect your partner. You don't have to be in love with someone to respect who they are as a person and care about their safety. If something comes up in your health or emotional life that affects your sex partner (like an STI or a new relationship protocol or boundary), the rules of consent (and common decency) demand you communicate that with them.

Respect yourself. If something changes and you need to renegotiate the terms of your relationship, do it. Don't suffer in silence pretending everything will work itself out. It rarely does.

One of the hardest things for folks in NSA relationships to navigate is when feelings take over. There's often pressure to keep it cool, aka "not have feelings." It's true that feelings can complicate things. It's also true that feelings are okay and trying to suppress them is guaranteed to make everything feel worse. Be open to the feelings. It's possible your NSA buddy may reciprocate. If they don't, you can have an honest conversation about what you both need to make the relationship feel okay going forward.

Respect the boundaries of NSA. As a person in an NSA arrangement, you are not allowed to tell the other person what they can and cannot do with their body. You don't get to tell them who to date, who to fuck, or anything. (This is generally true of all relationships, but is a particularly great feature of NSA.) You can express concern like anyone would, but the terms are clear: Everyone can fuck who they want, when they want, and you don't get a vote. So if you run into them at the club with another cutie on their arm, your jealousy is *your* business, not *their* problem.

NSA agreements can work great in short-term or long-term deals. They often end when one of you falls in love with someone else, develops a different relationship with different parameters, or just decides to call it quits for any reason. You're allowed to be tender and kind to that person, and you should definitely treat them like a human being.

Putting the "Us" in Anonymous

There's another, even more casual form of sex known simply as "anonymous." In anonymous sex arrangements, there's usually no meetup before and zero expectations besides "Come on up." Make no mistake, this kind of sex is the most risk-laden, which is precisely what draws some people to it. It can feel transgressive and edgy in a way that some people find super hot. Here are some ways to proceed:

Negotiate everything ahead of time. Anonymous doesn't mean no rules, it just means limited knowledge about each other's lives. Make it crystal clear what you're a yes to and what you're a no to. Let them know that if they violate your boundaries, you're out. Period.

PRO TIP

Some sex cultures rely on the context to set the rules. Bathhouses and some sex clubs, for instance, will often have posted rules or a monitor explain the expectations/regulations in a space to facilitate anonymous sex.

Meet them in neutral territory. On the street corner is good for this so they don't know your exact address, or a nearby bar or cafe, or in the hotel lobby. If you aren't feeling 100 percent down, tell them "thanks but no thanks."

Have a friend on call. Let your friend know when you're going to check in and be sure they can be trusted to swing by if you don't reach out at the designated time. Or better yet, enlist a beloved friend to be your bodyguard for the day and have them kick it outside. You might even include their role (with consent) in the fantasy for funsies.

Anonymous until proven otherwise. The agreement is anonymous, so expect fake names, and a blanket Don't Ask, Don't Tell policy. If you see them in the real world afterward, don't spill the beans about the details of your dirty dealings.

Have a hard out time. You could even gamify this by setting a timer or alarm clock to sound, after which they should be out the door. This will help you keep your word with your friend and give you an opportunity to check in with yourself to see if you're still having a good time.

Have plans afterward. If you're embarking on anonymous sex for the first time, it may be a good idea to have plans for afterward. Anonymous sex can be powerful shit, so plan to tend to your needs.

By definition, anonymous hookups are one-and-done situations. After that, they become more familiar. You decide if you want more action later, but the default setting is "Have a nice life."

Finding anonymous hookups can be like throwing spaghetti at the wall and seeing what sticks. Back in the Golden Age of the internet, Craigslist was the Road to El Dorado for anonymous sex-seekers. Nowadays, folks use apps such as Grindr and Tinder to generate possible hookups. Your success rate will likely rely on your micro culture. Queer men looking for other queer men, for instance, generally have an easier time finding hookups than straight men looking for women. C'est la bang.

Booty Booty Booty!

Ah, the noble booty call. They've been around since time immemorial, perhaps beginning with the booty cry across the canyon, evolving into the booty carrier pigeon, then the booty letter, and the booty telegram, before arriving at our most recent ancestor, the booty telephone call. Nowadays, a couple of emojis in a text can do the trick. Luckily, while technology has changed, the etiquette has remained pretty consistent. Here are the Five Rules of Booty Calls:

1 **It's only a booty call if you've *already* had sex together.** As a general rule, don't offer a short-notice, low-maintenance bang session to someone you haven't banged yet, or at least talked about it with. That's just tacky. The one exception? If you met them via an app or website designed for getting laid, NSA-style. Then, though, it's technically a hookup and not a booty call.

2 **Be clear with your intentions.** If you invite someone over promising dinner and a movie, but all you're gunning for is sex, be honest about it. At least let them know before they come over that "eating in" was a euphemism.

3 **Don't double dip.** You send a text to Hottie #1. How long do you wait before you text Hottie #2? While there's no science to it, it's poor form to be impatient. Give Hottie #1 ample time to respond before moving on to the next. An hour is a good rule of thumb. Maybe they were at a movie?

4 **Honor your word.** Don't make them jump through a bunch of hoops to get into your bed. Are you meeting at their place or yours? When? Best be there then, kiddo. Beckoning a sweetie to your place and then losing track of time at the bar is a great way to make sure you don't get repeat business, and worse, earn yourself a bad reputation.

5 **Sleepovers are optional, but should be negotiated beforehand.** Kicking someone to the curb when there aren't easy and safe options to get home in the wee hours isn't cool. But it's also presumptuous to expect to sleep over if it wasn't decided already. So talk it through. If your bang buddy needs to sleep over but you're not keen on sharing your bed, make sure they have another comfy option in your place.

Slumber Party!

Hosting a sleepover? How fun! I'll grab my sleeping bag and some nail polishes!
Oh, not that kind of sleepover? Even better.

If you're in the position of snuggling a sweetie in your bed, you have my congratulations. Here are some ways to win the sleepover game:

Have safer sex supplies. The answer to the age-old riddle "Who brings the condoms to a booty call?" is: *everyone.* If you're having sex, bring the gear you need to keep yourself and your partners safe. There's no excuse if you're the one hosting. Have condoms and lube available so your partner feels comfortable.

Make sure your room is comfortable. Make sure you have enough blankets and pillows for the both of you to sleep comfortably. Have a cat? Consider sexiling Mr. Snuffles for the night so you can give other pussies a chance to enjoy themselves. Think in terms of what would make a new person feel safe and comfortable in your room.

> I once hooked up with a guy who loved cold rooms. I didn't mind it at all until I "slept" over. It wasn't really sleeping, though, because while he snoozed beside me, I was curled up, shivering under the single sheet on the bed, beneath an open window I couldn't figure out how to close. Oh, did I mention it was January in Ohio? I didn't get any sleep that night, contemplating how hard it would be to walk home at three a.m. through the snow if I couldn't find both my socks. Not good. You can bet that was the last time I answered his booty call.

Provide basic creature comforts. Bring them water or make sure they know how to get it. Are you a snorer? Have earplugs. No curtains? An eye mask is a lovely thing to offer. And of course, let them know where they can plug in their phone.

To cuddle, or not to cuddle? If you just banged or something like it, talking about cuddling should be a nonissue. Regardless, it's nice to bring up. Like being the big spoon? Can't sleep with anyone touching you at all? Say so to avoid hurt feelings.

Communicate about morning stuff. Gotta get to work at seven? Wondering if they prefer coffee or tea? Let them know before you fall asleep so everyone feels like they're on the same page. You're not obligated to let them stay in your place after you've left, but if you're up and out early, give them the chance to emotionally prepare for a six a.m. alarm. Some folks like to rack up bonus points by greeting their bang buddy with morning pancakes. If you want to add that arrow to your quiver, by all means do. Otherwise, coffee/tea and a sweet thank-you is usually sufficient (and appreciated).

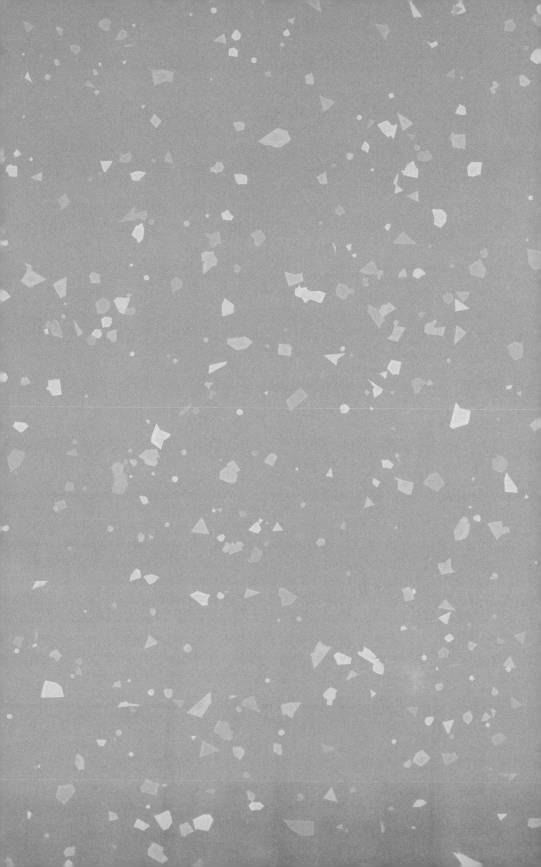

Tech Support

In this modern era of boning, many of your interactions with sex partners will be online in some way. In fact, sometimes it seems like cell phones were designed to get people laid. By the time this book gets from my brain into your hands, there will probably be at least four new dating apps, three new social media crazes, and countless new ways to psychologically torture each other. Tech can make life simpler, but it also adds complications. See, humans have evolved a whole set of tools that technology doesn't always facilitate—things such as eye contact, tone of voice, facial expressions, touch, and even scent. So when you flirt via chat, it's likely you're not picking up on the cues you might otherwise notice in real life.

To be clear, this tech is *effective*. A recent study showed 40 percent of hetero-paired couples met online, and nearly 60 percent of same-sex couples did. It also opens up new avenues for sexy interactions. Let's tour the etiquette of sexy action at a distance.

Finger My App

Luckily, the rules of dating apps are pretty similar to the rules of IRL: Be upfront about who you are and what you're looking for. Realize most people are going to judge you based on the pictures, so make sure they're in focus and accurately represent you. Consider having a friend of the gender you're seeking review your profile. If you're a certain kind of geek, you can even gamify this and do A/B tests with different pictures and profile info.

If you swipe right on each other, congrats! Spend a little time getting to know each other on the app first before moving forward. Most apps have a block feature, so if things take a weird turn, staying in the app means your flirt-friend won't have your personal info. The first interaction is often the hardest. Gather clues by rereading their profile and looking through their pictures, then say something that's relevant to what they shared. A "Hi" or "U up?" is unlikely to garner you quality results. Instead, ask a question or share something you noticed in their profile that interested you.

If after chatting it seems like you're compatible, make plans to meet up in real life. Do it sooner rather than later. A little flirting is fine, but don't get stuck in the Chasm of Faceless Sexting. You need to meet the person and see if you're *actually* compatible, not just virtually.

Here are some rules for first dates:

→ **Keep it public.** Make plans to meet somewhere other than either of your homes and in neutral territory (i.e., not your daily coffee shop). Also, take a tip from an Oregonian: most hikes are *not* public.

→ **Keep it contained.** Have loose plans after the date to ensure you have an out. If things are going *really* well, you can always cancel your later plans or, better yet, keep that juicy anticipation going until next time.

→ **If they seem like a good fit, make a second date.** If not, thank them for their time and let them know you're not feeling it. You can do this in person (best) or later via the app (less great, but better than ghosting).

Above all, remember that dating is a pain in the ass for many people. It requires money, time, and a general game attitude. Don't ghost, try to honor your commitments, and if you're not feeling a spark with an otherwise decent person, be gracious and let them off the hook.

PRO TIP

It's no secret that the internet/world is filled with some major assholes. Dating and hookup sites seem to attract the worst of the worst. Minimize your suffering by keeping your private info private until you've built a foundation of trust. Screenshot abuse and report it to the app. You may be saving other people from gross behavior in the future.

Sexting

Flirting via text is one of my favorite sexy-time activities. It's lower pressure than flirting IRL, you can take your time, revise and edit, and even call for backup when you're stuck. For the less verbally inclined among us, though, it can feel intimidating.

Once you've got those digits, here's how to proceed:

Get permission to flirt. If you're not sure the object of your affection is game for some hot flirting action, or if you want to make sure flirting fits within the parameters of their existing relationship(s), check in first.

> "I want to tell you about the hot dream I had about you last night. Would you like that?"

> "I've been having some naughty thoughts since we last hooked up. Wanna hear them?"

> "You are super cute and I like flirting with you. Can I keep doing it?"

Escalate with care. Pay attention to the tone that's been set by your interactions so far. Is it playful and sweet? Filthy? Somewhere in between? Note what's working and tiptoe toward the more sexual if it feels right.

Reveal, don't demand. It's okay to ask for a sexy fantasy from your flirt-friend, but it's a good idea to establish trust by revealing intimate aspects of yourself more often.

> "I woke up thinking about how much I want to kiss you."

> "I had a fun idea I'd like to try next time we see each other. May I share?"

> "I have an elaborate bondage fantasy starring you. Want to hear it?"

Understand lag time, but let them know if there will be a long delay. You will likely establish a rhythm with your flirt-friend. Some folks keep their phones on them all the time, while others check their messages sporadically. While the lack of required immediacy is one of text-flirting's best parts, it can also exacerbate anxiety or insecurity, particularly if there's no clear pattern to when and how you respond. If it's going to take you a long time to respond to a text, try to give them a heads-up. Transparency is key.

Coyness, not confusion. It's okay to play it cool, but fostering confusion is manipulative. Don't hang back from responding to a date request just to play hard to get. Don't withhold your feelings or answers to direct questions just to manifest an air of mystery. You're more likely to foster frustration and resentment. Be kind. Handle people's hearts with care.

Assume good intent. This is just a generally helpful life rule, but it goes extra for texting. Ever notice how texts don't include tone of voice or eye contact? This is how tech removes context clues and flattens discourse, making it much easier to misinterpret the intent of the person you're talking with.

DO'S AND DON'TS OF SENDING PHOTO SEXTS

Who doesn't love getting a sexy picture from a sexy friend? Sharing pics can up the energy in a text flirtation, but they come with their own etiquette. Here are some do's and don'ts for snapping that ass:

DO ask permission. Don't just send a picture of your genitals without asking. You can ask first in a flirty way: "Just got out of the shower and looking fly. Can I send a pic?" Make sure you get a yes from the person before you send any nekkid shots. If they say no, respect it and don't read too much into it. They may have a work cell phone or nosy kids, or they may just prefer to imagine the sexy.

DO remember that sexts are forever. The world is full of horror stories of folks being hurt by pictures they've sent to an ex. Don't send anything you aren't okay with living on in the interminable memory of the internet. And yes, internet security being what it is, the government can totally see your junk. That is a fact. If that freaks you out, don't send the pics. Also, if you're underage, play it safe and stick to text! You could be prosecuted for "distributing child porn" even if you're sending pictures of *yourself*.

DON'T send pictures if you don't want to. And don't let anyone guilt you into sending pictures you aren't comfortable with. Your body, your choice.

DO keep your face out of frame if that feels better for you. It may not protect you from the government totally seeing your junk, or shitty exes saying, "That is totally my ex's junk," but it does add some deniability.

DO know that words are good, too. If you don't want to send booty shots, why not some choice dirty talk? Send a couple lines of things you want to do to your sweetie the next time you see them, or choice memories from the last time you were together. Yum.

> My partner loves sending me nudes when I'm traveling. It helps keep the romance alive. It's also really awkward to get a big ol' dick pic when I'm, for instance, getting settled on a plane. So, if you're feeling the urge to send some filth to your flame, ask if they'd prefer a picture or some text. It's good practice to mix it up and helps avoid embarrassing seatmate situations.

DO'S AND DON'TS OF RECEIVING SEXTS

If you're on the receiving end of some sexy smut from a sweetie, congratulations! Let it fill your heart and loins with joy. Next:

DO be gracious. A single heart-eyed emoji doesn't cut it. Thank them for the nice picture, tell them what it made you think of, and reciprocate if that works for you. Let them know how sexy/beautiful/fuckable you think they look.

DON'T go all radio silence. They can't see you blush. Say something.

DO delete them when asked. Yes, every single one. Yes, from everywhere.

DON'T share them! Respect the people who share their bodies with you! Don't violate their privacy by showing the pictures to anyone else. If you want to show the picture to your bestie, ask permission from the sender first. For the love of all that is good in the world, DON'T POST ON THE INTERNET. Not only is it unethical, it's also illegal. Revenge porn is a crime and a form of sexual assault. Don't fucking do it.

* * *

Okay, so now that we've laid the ground rules, what makes a good sext?

→ **Know your audience.** Is your sweetie fond of your booty? Or maybe your lips? Do they like a little left to the imagination? Or do they want to see it ALL? Knowing what your partner likes will help you figure out a good shot. One person's pout is another one's crotch shot.

→ **Framing, lighting, and angle.** Photography is an art, so why not treat it like one? Pay attention to what's in frame, and what's not. Sometimes cutting off the shot *juuuuuust* at the edge of the goods can be superbly titillating. Consider using a mirror or a selfie stick to improve your ability to reach the right spots. Bright ambient light is good for cell phone snaps, but it can also reveal a little too much sometimes. Play with light and shadow to upgrade your smut to art.

→ **Authenticity is a virtue.** While filters and photo editing can make you feel extra cute, go easy on the special effects.

→ **Timing.** Away from your sweetie for a while? It can be fun to re-up their gooey feelings for you by sending a sext in between dates, or when you know they've had a tough day. Consider sending a sext to let them know you just masturbated thinking of them. Depending on their sense of humor, use caution when sexting during business hours, lest your goods make an accidental appearance in the conference room.

Reach Out and Touch Someone

Phone sex is essentially dirty talk plus distance. This distance means you can make up pretty much anything and you won't have to try hard to suspend your disbelief (as opposed to in real life sex when saying, "I'm flogging your ass" while you're tweaking their nipple can create some cognitive dissonance.) There are three main dirty talk flavors: real-time description, recollection, and fantasy weaving. If you're just dipping your toes into the dirty talk waters, real-time description and recollection are good places to start.

Real-time description is just saying what's happening. Simple. So if you're on the phone, touching yourself, you describe how you're touching yourself, how it feels, and perhaps what you're thinking about. Here are some examples:

> "I've got my favorite dildo in my pussy and feeling it hit my G-spot."

> "I'm tugging on my balls and imagining it's your hand."

Easy peasy, sexy teasy.

Recollection is great if you have a sexual history with your phone mate already. Simply describe a hot time you had together:

> "Remember that hot tub in Aspen? I sat on your lap and grinded on you until I came?"

> "I'm thinking about that time in the movie theater. The way your fingers crept into my jeans . . ."

If you don't have a sexual history with this person, or none of the stories are inspiring, you can still use your past as inspiration. Maybe describe a hot masturbatory session you had or a porn you watched. If your partner is cool with you talking about sex you've had with other people, those stories can be delightfully juicy to share with a new paramour.

Fantasy weaving is what most people think about when it comes to dirty talk. This can include role-play, fantastical scenarios, or just what you want to do to/with your phone buddy the next time you're in the same place. It can also be the hardest, since it's essentially filthy improv. It works like improv, too—you need a setting and a concept:

"But Captain, you promised I could go on shore with the other boys if I finished my chores! What else can I possibly do?"

"You're going to pick me up from the airport and take me straight to the grungiest motel you can find . . ."

"Then the dragon mother screeches and says, 'To secure my fortune, you must prove you have the greatest cock in all of Alorthien!'"

You can also give your partner a sexy prompt:

"What will do you do to me when I visit next month?"

"What are you imagining I'm doing to you right now?"

"Tell me about the time that . . ."

Power dynamics can be integrated into phone sex to delightful effect. For the dominant sorts, consider:

"I want to listen to you fuck yourself, but don't come until I tell you to."

"As soon as we hang up, I want you to send me a picture of your sweet, pliant mouth."

And for the submissive types:

> "What do you want me to do to myself, sir?"

> "May I please put the dildo inside me?"

Don't forget your voice! When someone is giving you yummy fantasy fodder, it's polite to offer sounds of sexy acknowledgment. A little moan or giggle here and there helps keep the flow going. If you're talking to get each other off, give your partner a heads-up about how close you are to coming. It's awkward to have another warrior-knight stride into the love cave two minutes after your partner is done. Trust me on that one.

SIT ON MY FACETIME

The tips for phone dirty talk apply to video-chatting as well, with the added benefit of getting to see your partner's O-face. If you're going to partake, make sure you have decent Wi-Fi. There's nothing more frustrating than frozen video when you're getting juicy. Good lighting is a must. The grainy blue-on-black look isn't sexy, so add a warm lamp to make sure your skin looks good. Also, consider your frame. Do you want the camera to show maximum skin or do you want to leave most of it to the imagination? Using a Bluetooth mouse and external camera can help you get the angles just right.

Don't record without permission! In most states in the United States it's illegal to record a phone call without disclosing you're doing it. That's why when you call a customer service line, a robot says, "This call may be recorded for training purposes." So don't record the call unless you tell them and they say, "Hell yes!" And if you're under eighteen, don't record yourself at all.

Partnered Pleasure

Stereotypes about gender differences regarding casual sex are greatly over-stated. Studies show regardless of gender, most adults enjoy the prospect of casual sex. For vulva-owners and folks on the trans spectrum, however, while we may *want* to have sex, it can be harder for us to find physical pleasure in hookups. Whether it's because we're not as familiar with the working of our bodies or that society doesn't prize our pleasure as much as cis dudes', I don't know. (Actually, I *do* know. It's both.) These factors contribute to what's known as the Orgasm Gap.

The Orgasm Gap

The Orgasm Gap refers to the relative ease and therefore frequency cis men have in achieving orgasm versus cis women during hetero, partnered sex. There's a lot to unpack here already, but first let's acknowledge that this gap is based solely on studies of cis, hetero sex. So for simplicity's sake, in this sec-tion only, I'm speaking directly to cis men and cis women.

There are plenty of things to blame for the Orgasm Gap, but there are two big culprits. The first one is obvious: during penis-vagina sex, the penis gets stimu-lated, but much of the clitoris does not. While the penis is the primary pleasure organ in cis guys, the vagina is *not* the main pleasure organ in cis women. So the main way straight people have sex leaves a woman's primary pleasure organ out in the cold. This is like if every time a straight couple had sex, the woman only fingered a guy's ass and ignored his cock. Like, sure, the guy might enjoy it. And sure, he may even come from it. But it's kind of missing a *biiiiiig* part of pleasure.

The less obvious but equally important reason for the Orgasm Gap is a seri-ous lack of interest in women's pleasure. This comes from treating women as holes to penetrate instead of human beings to give pleasure to. Our entire cul-ture is to blame for this. We treat "scoring" as getting your dick wet, no matter if she enjoyed it, or even liked you. We consider it more of a success to get a begrudging two minutes of humping instead of forty minutes of intense, con-nected makeouts. This has lots to do with our shitty sex-education system. When we talk all about diseases and pregnancy, and nothing about pleasure and desire, it's no wonder so many of us feel clumsy and uninformed.

Here's a fun fact: Lesbians have orgasms 86 percent of the time they have partnered sex, compared to 65 percent for straight women.[1] Sure, lesbians might better know the terrain, but they also have a wider understanding of what "counts" as sex. If you're a dude who has sex with women, here's what you can learn from your Sapphic sisters, and close the gap:

Understand anatomy. You can't drive to the amusement park if you don't know the way. Learn about genitals and how they respond to touch. Read *Girl Sex 101* and Sheri Winston's *Women's Anatomy of Desire* for a full primer on vulva pleasure and things to do to your lady and/or parts. (See page 270 for more suggestions.)

There's no such thing as foreplay. It's all part of the sex. Oral sex, fingers, breast play—it's all sex. So don't treat them like boxes to check off on your way to the "real thing."

Outercourse. Women are not just holes to be filled. Once you understand how her body is put together, you can bring pleasure to the rest of her. Unless she requests otherwise, focus on her clitoris, where eight thousand nerve endings are waiting for attention.

While we're on the topic: Did you know the clitoris is made up of erectile tissue? In fact, pound for pound, inch for inch, the clitoris has the *same amount of erectile tissue as the penis*. Read that again. Yeah. Most of the clit, however, is on the *inside*. The clitoris and the penis have a whole lot in common. One main difference, however, is how long the clitoris takes to get erect. Some research shows it can take between twenty minutes to a full hour for the clit to get fully aroused. This doesn't mean your partner isn't feeling anything until an hour in, but it *does* emphasize why "foreplay," anticipation, and luxurious timelines all help her get *more* excited.

Slow. The. Fuck. Down. Some folks are so eager to get to the penetration part of the game, they completely ignore the rest of their partner's body. If you go too fast, you're not giving your partner enough time to warm up and feel good.

Be a generous lover. Partnered sex is about the joy of giving and sharing pleasure, not just taking it. Humans aren't sex toys (unless you negotiated that one *hard* up front, but . . . that's a different book). Cultivate pleasure in giving. Take joy in the sounds they make and the things they request. Be willing to learn and invite their feedback. Endeavor to be, as Dan Savage says, Good, Giving, and Game.

Professional tools create professional results. Sex toys aren't just for solo sex. While some people may get nervous sharing space with a vibrator, those concerns are often dispelled when they see what great results toys offer. Use a vibrator with your partner or get another kind of toy to explore together, like a buttplug. Some folks might consider that kinky, to which I say, "Right on!" If you're having casual sex, ideally, you'll feel free explore all sorts of fun things.

Deprioritize orgasm. I know, that sounds contradictory. Here's the thing though: lots of people attach their ego to how many times they can "make" their partner come, putting way too much pressure on everyone to "perform" during sex. While I appreciate the magnanimity, it can create a feedback loop of pressure and anxiety, which contradicts a good time. So instead of making it all about orgasm . . .

Prioritize *pleasure*. Treat your partner as a whole person, paying attention to their physical and emotional comfort, and dedicate time and attention to sharing pleasure. Encourage your partner to breathe and relax, and your focus is on just making their body feel good.

TRANSGASMS

There's not much research on orgasms and trans people, but much of the same advice applies, with the added challenges of dysphoria and hormones. If you and/or your lover are trans, here are some ways you can help achieve orgasm together.

Honor their body. Many trans folks have pain or anxiety attached to sex, which makes pleasure harder to come by. Use specific and loving language and touch to create a space where you both can relax and receive pleasurable touch.

Respect cycles. Everyone has hormones and everyone experiences hormonal cascades and cycles. Hormones taken in pills or injections, though, can offer the opportunity for a bit more predictability than innate hormones. After taking a dose of hormones, some people can experience rushes of emotions or sensations that abate as their bodies metabolize the hormones. For instance, some trans girls find their nipples become sensitive soon after they take their hormones. An attentive lover might consider this useful information. If you're the one taking hormones, consider keeping a journal to track how sensations and emotions flow through you after taking your dose.

Be patient. Patience means being okay living inside the complexity of people and bodies. What feels good one day may be painful (physically or emotionally) the next. Being patient means treating this as just another aspect of being human. If you or your partner have new genitals or a new chest, you may need to spend some time figuring out how all the new bits work. Parts that once felt great may be numb, and parts that once were painful can be great sources of joy. It may take some time to relearn how everything works.

Be creative. Say it with me: Every. Body. Is. Different. It doesn't matter how you identify, what feels good to one person may not to another. Yeah, many sex books (mine included!) try to give you tips that tend to work well for most people, but that doesn't mean a technique is gonna work for every person at every moment. Sexual creativity is a virtue. It'll help you in the long run. Be open, be malleable, and be willing to try new things in pursuit of pleasure.

* * *

Regardless of gender or orientation, we can all do our part to mind the Orgasm Gap, by educating ourselves about pleasure (both our own and our partners') and advocating for ourselves.

Masturbate. Your pleasure is in, well, your hands. Just like you shouldn't rely on a partner to feed you, you shouldn't have to rely on them to get you off, either. That's *your* job. Clock some time exploring so you can learn what works and then give your partners the cheat codes to your goods.

Advocate and communicate. Once you know what you like, share those things, verbally.

Expand your idea of sex. For plenty of people of all orientations and identities, conventional penis-in-vagina (P/V) sex isn't all that exciting. They may prefer oral or anal or impact play or power exchange or mutual masturbation or the bajillion other ways humans like to fool around together. If P/V isn't exciting or possible for you, chuck it and play in other ways.

Be a selfish lover. If you have a difficult orgasm or are a chronic people-pleaser, you may need to give yourself more permission to receive. If your partner says they want to give you pleasure, believe them. If they say they get as much joy out of going down on you (or whatever) as you do, trust them. Letting someone give you joy, or giving them the opportunity to try to "crack the code" of your orgasm, can be wonderful fun for everyone.

Lend a hand. You are allowed, and in fact *encouraged*, to touch yourself during sex. It can be super hot to watch your partner play with themselves. So encourage your partner to touch themselves, and don't be afraid to do it yourself.

Upgrade. If you are sleeping with people who don't care to put in the effort for your pleasure, especially after communicating what you want, find new partners. There are plenty of eager and generous lovers in this world. Reward them with your time and energy.

Detailed sex technique is outside the scope of this book, but luckily there are dozens of books and videos to look to. An overarching piece of advice: Consider porn an entertainment medium, not an educational one. The people in porn are putting on a show, not teaching technique. For actual sexual pleasure info, scoot on over to page 270 and stuff your brain.

Curiosity and Play

Recently, I was in bed with a new sweetie who expressed a little delighted shock at how much I giggled during sex. He said, "I've never been with someone who has so much *fun* during sex before."

Sex doesn't always have to be a laugh riot. There are plenty of times when it should be anything but silly. However, it's helpful to remember that sex has a strong relationship to play. Children learn about one another by interacting, trying things, and seeing what works. So do adults. We just have different kinds of toys.

Casual sex is the perfect playground for exploring the fun, the goofy, and the odd. If you think your sex could benefit from a bit more silliness and joy, here are some ways to foster it:

Acknowledge that bodies are weird. They make weird sounds and smells. When sweaty bodies touch they sometimes make that hilarious fart sound. Sometimes you'll have a hard time getting hard, wet, calm, ready, and all the things. We're all just sentient meat sacks making our way in the world. Acknowledge your body plays by its own rules sometimes and sometimes those rules are wacky as hell.

Your mind is probably weird, too, at least a little. I used to think I was pretty normal. Basic, even. Then I started getting intimate with people who delighted in how odd and goofy I was, in bed and out. It's true that the more comfortable we tend to get with people, the more willing we are to be our true selves, and sometimes those selves are *weeeeeird*. When it comes to casual sex it's a good idea to *lead with the weird*. Yes, you'll scare some people off. The ones who stick around are usually the kind of quality humans you want in your life.

Keep an open mind. Sometimes your partner will reveal something that takes you by surprise. A fetish, perhaps, or a fantasy or a technique that turns their crank. When this happens, you have a choice to make: roll with it or stop.

It's okay to have a moment of adjustment if you get caught off guard. However, being thrown isn't a license to shame. So keep your negative opinions to yourself. If you need to take some time to decide whether you're up for exploring something with your partner, take the time you need. If you need more information about how they'd like to explore it, ask for elucidation.

Creativity is a virtue. Odds are you're going to encounter a sex partner who has limitations you'll both have to work with. The good news is restriction fosters creativity. You often find wells of inspiration and energy when your usual vectors are closed. Look for the middle ground and see how much fun you can have there.

Gamify your sex. That same lover who delighted in my playfulness was surprised the first time he spanked me. Reader, I laughed. Hearty, belly laughs. "That's not what I was going for," he said. "Well, spank me harder until I stop laughing," I replied. I'm happy to report we both got what we were looking for in that moment. Sometimes a little competition in the spirit of good sportsmanship can create fun for everyone.

Sexual Health

Every day we make choices that affect our health: what we eat, where we live, how we get around, how we spend our time. For every choice we make, someone has opinions. So many opinions.

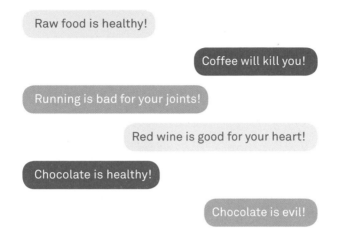

Raw food is healthy!

Coffee will kill you!

Running is bad for your joints!

Red wine is good for your heart!

Chocolate is healthy!

Chocolate is evil!

And on and on and on. Here's *my* opinion:

Your body is your own and you can use and/or abuse it any way you choose. I believe most people are aware of the consequences of their choices but are willing to hedge their bets. Seriously, do you know any cigarette smoker who *doesn't* know smoking causes cancer? Probably not. But you likely still know smokers. Similarly, American football is *wildly* dangerous, sending hundreds of thousands of people to the emergency room every year. Skiing, horseback riding, cycling, surfing—these things aren't safe. But safety isn't the point. Sports enthusiasts choose to take on the consequences of their actions, or they choose to ignore the facts and live in the moment. Whatever anyone's reason for anything, it doesn't matter. What matters is what *you* choose, with eyes wide open.

Every choice has consequences. The question is, which consequences are you most comfortable living with? Celibacy has consequences. So does promiscuity. Monogamy has consequences, as does nonmonogamy. For some folks, abstaining from sex and thereby lowering risk of things such as STIs, pregnancy, and unwanted emotions is totally worth the lack of sexual connection with people. To others, the risks of living a slutty life are worth it to experience free self-expression and the deep intimacy of sexual connection.

Understanding the consequences of your choices is the first step of what's known as **risk assessment**. In terms of sex, risk assessment means (1) understanding the nature and likelihood of an unwanted consequence of a sexual choice, and (2) the effect of that consequence on yourself and others. Some such consequences are STIs, pregnancy, emotional harm, community disruption, and good old-fashioned drama.

"Safe" is relative. Decide what safety means to you, and then design your boundaries and protocols accordingly. The riskiest sex of all is the kind where *no one talks about it*. So talk about it, and insist your hookup buddies do, too.

— Casual Sex Risk Assessment —

Here's how to conduct your own risk assessment. At first this may feel cumbersome. Once you get good at knowing yourself it will become second nature.

1   **Arm yourself with knowledge.** Understand how the risky stuff works. Learn about STIs and their prevention, contraception, and your own emotional state. Get a grasp on how social hierarchies affect sexual choices. For instance, it's clear that in hetero sex, women bear the brunt of risk in terms of pregnancy, STIs, and potential for abuse. If you live in a place that prohibits abortion, casual sex may carry significant, life-altering risks. If you're an out queer, some of your sex partners might not be as out as you are or have a support system. Once you understand how society makes some people safer than others, you can understand how risk affects everyone involved. Certain sexy-time activities are risker than others, too. Impact play, anal, bondage, dirty talk—they all carry their own risks. If you're enthusiastic about any forms of kink/BDSM, educate yourself on their risks and how to minimize potential harms to yourself and your partners.

2   **Prioritize the risks.** Every activity has risks. Some will be more nerve-wracking to you than others. Some folks will be super concerned about pregnancy, others will be worried about disclosing their gender identity. Some folks will be worried about HIV, others will be worried about exacerbation of chronic pain. Once you are aware of all the risks, prioritize those that are most pressing to you.

3   **Tackle the risks in order of priority.** Many risks are simple to manage. Worried about HIV? Use condoms and consider getting a prescription for pre-exposure prophylactic (PrEP). Worried about pregnancy? Get yourself reliable birth control! Others can be more ineffable: things such as shame, challenging communications, and trauma. Do what you need to do (whether it's therapy, shoring up your friendships, or whatever) to tackle the risks so you can feel safer engaging in your chosen behaviors.

Sometimes you won't see a risk until you're experiencing it. Do your best to navigate on the fly, and learn what you can from it. Soon enough, you'll walk through the world knowing which risks are reasonable to you and which aren't, so you can make the choice that feels best.

STIs and Safer Sex

While the rest of this book helps you navigate emotional stakes, this section will teach you about the physical ones, namely STIs. Sexually transmitted infections are viruses, parasites, and bacterial infections that can be transmitted through sexual contact. While sex is a good way to transmit all sorts of things (like the common cold, for instance).

THE DIFFERENT TYPES OF STIS AND HOW ARE THEY TRANSMITTED

STIs are so-named because they are *only* or *most likely* transmitted via sexual contact. Some STIs are transmitted through blood, some through genital fluids (precum, semen, vaginal secretions, and "female" ejaculate), some through saliva, and some through skin/skin contact.

HIV: The big scary one, human immunodeficiency viruses (HIV), should be on your radar if you enjoy blood play, or penis/vagina (P/V) or penis/anus (P/A) sex. Despite all the horror stories, HIV is avoidable if you play responsibly. Use a barrier (either an internal or external condom) and don't share needles (this goes for injectable drugs, piercing play, and DIY tattoos).

Gloves and dental dams/condoms can add extra protection. The rate of transmission is low for oral sex, but it's often better to go overboard with protection than panic the next morning.

If you think you've been exposed, visit your local clinic or hospital and ask for a PEP (post-exposure prophylactic), which can protect you from contracting the virus, even if it made its way into your body.

Consider getting a prescription for a PrEP such as Truvada, a daily pill that prevents HIV transmission. The drug has proven to be about 98 percent effective at preventing the contraction of HIV after exposure.[1] People with an undetectable viral load can't infect others, but if you're sleeping with someone who's HIV positive, it's still a fine idea to take PrEP for added safety measure.

HPV: Doctors test for the human papillomavirus (HPV) with a cervical Pap smear. Some strains (about thirteen of the thirty varieties of the virus) can lead to cervical cancer. Other strains can cause genital or anal warts. The rest are often inert, just hanging out but not causing symptoms or discomfort, or eventually fought off by your immune system. The vaccine Gardasil 9 prevents about 90 percent of the cancer-causing strains,[2] and may also prevent transmission of warts. All genders can get Gardasil 9, though the age range is limited based on FDA approval. For sexually active folks, getting the vaccine is a great way to reduce the risk of contracting and spreading HPV. I strongly recommend talking to your doctor about it.

The best precautions against HPV are to avoid direct genital/genital contact and don't penetrate yourself with anything that penetrated your partner unless you wash it well and/or switch out the barrier.

Hepatitis: Hepatitis is an inflammation of the liver. Heps A, B, and C have similar symptoms though they're caused by different viruses. Hep A is spread by ingesting infected feces (as can happen with rimming), Hep B by ingesting infected blood or other body fluids (like semen or vaginal fluid), and Hep C is transmitted by ingesting infected blood (such as through cunnilingus during menstruation). Heps A and B have vaccines, and many people are vaccinated as children. Hep C doesn't have a vaccine yet. The key to avoiding or managing hepatitis is knowing your status and the status of your partners. Get vaccinated if you haven't been already, and when in doubt, use barriers for all oral sex, as well as genital/genital contact.

PRO TIP

Menstrual fluid is mostly blood. So it can put you at risk for Heps B and C. Be cautious of eating out your partner during Shark Week. Want to go to town even when it's a-flowin? Use barriers (like a dental dam), use a tampon/menstrual cup, get tested, and get vaccinated.

Herpes: If you think you don't have herpes, you're probably wrong. Fifty-eight percent of all Americans and Canadians have HSV-1 (most often oral) herpes. For Europeans it's between 65 and 87 percent. About one in five Americans has HSV-2 (most commonly genital herpes).[3]

Most people are asymptomatic, which means they don't have outbreaks and may never know they have the virus. Doctors don't usually test for it unless you get an outbreak, and standard STI panels don't include the test either. Like warts, the virus just hangs out in your body not doing much until you're sick, stressed, or otherwise immunosuppressed.

While this may freak you out, the good news is herpes is really a dermatological problem. It can cause embarrassing and/or painful sores on your lips or genitals, but it's not going to kill you, and it may not even cause discomfort. Unless you're immunosuppressed or expecting to give birth when you're having an outbreak, it's not something to freak out about.

Herpes is spread via skin-to-skin contact, like kissing, and evidence shows you can contract it even when the carrier isn't having an outbreak. The best approach is to avoid direct contact with anyone's sores, ask your partner if they get cold sores and tell them if you do, take care of your body and immune system, and use barriers for oral sex if you're worried about genital herpes.

PRO TIP

Herpes is *common*. So stop making jokes about it as though it's the worst thing that can happen to someone. Yes, it can be uncomfortable and embarrassing, but a big part of that is jerks mocking folks with herpes like they're unclean lepers. Grow up, people.

Chlamydia, gonorrhea, and syphilis: Bacterial infections such as chlamydia, gonorrhea, and syphilis can be treated with antibiotics. Some clinicians are concerned about the rise of an antibiotic-resistant strain of gonorrhea, but as of this writing it's still totally treatable. Barriers can protect against transmission.

Trichomoniasis: A parasite that's transmitted via sexual contact, trichomoniasis causes 3.7 million infections each year.[4] It's treated with antibiotics. Symptoms are rarer in people with penises, so they can be carriers without knowing it. You can get trich from fluid exchange, like oral sex or genital/genital contact. You can protect yourself by using barriers for oral sex and genital/genital sex.

GETTING TESTED

All of this info is great, but it doesn't mean much unless you know your status. Many STIs don't cause symptoms until they've progressed, and these are things you want to nip in the bud. Your primary care physician, urgent care facility, or gynecologist can administer the tests. Just say you want an STI screening. Insurance usually covers a standard panel (HIV, HPV, hepatitis, chlamydia, trichomoniasis, gonorrhea, and syphilis). To find the free and cheap testing centers near you, visit Hivtest.cdc.gov.

It's okay to be nervous, but what's more important is learning your status. Blissful ignorance doesn't last long. Most STIs are treatable and manageable, but only if you catch them early.

WHAT DOES AN STI TEST LOOK LIKE?

A complete STI test usually consists of (1) a blood draw, (2) a urine test, and (3) a Pap smear (for cervix-owners). Some places also do oral, anal, throat, and/or urethral swabs. You can ask what the test will entail before you go to the clinic. Many clinics have drop-in screenings, anonymous or confidential services, as well as treatment and education programs. Most LGBTQ+ centers and Planned Parenthoods offer testing or referrals regardless of your gender or sexuality.

Some results are available immediately, as with rapid HIV tests. Sometimes your samples have to be sent away for testing, and you get the results by phone. Any reputable clinic will give you all the info you need to get your results and ensure your privacy.

WHEN SHOULD I GET TESTED?

Get tested as soon as you start being sexually active. Then, get tested after each new partner, after any risky encounters (e.g., unbarriered sex or disclosure of an STI by a partner), if you have any odd symptoms, or every three to eight months, depending on how sexually active you are.

SAFER SEX PROTOCOL

A safer sex protocol is what you need to feel both emotionally and physically safe in bed. Everyone's protocols are different and often change based on relationship status, your partner's needs and disclosures, your general health and well-being, and your preferred modes of sexual play.

Design your protocol so it's in alignment with your sense of safety and integrity. For instance, you might be okay with hand sex or toys for a one-night stand, but you only have oral sex with people you're serious about. Or, you might not play with anyone until they've been tested.

BARRIERS

Barriers minimize fluid exchange and, short of abstinence, they're one of the best ways to mitigate your STI risk. Typical barriers are condoms, dental dams, and gloves. These all come in both latex and nitrile. Check in with your partner if they have a latex allergy before you use a barrier.

External condoms are what most people think of when they think of condoms. They're a thin latex or nitrile sheath designed to cover an erect penis before penetrative sex. They're cheap, they're effective, and they changed the motherfucking world. But they're not just for peens! You can use condoms on dildos or vibrators to keep them clean and make them easier to share. There's a huge variety of condoms on the market, ranging in size, texture, color, etc. If you're looking for condoms on the cheap (or on the free), check out your local LGBTQ+ center or Planned Parenthood.

Internal condoms are usually called "female condoms." They're larger, looser condoms that go inside the receiver. Because of this, they can be inserted before sex and don't rely on an erection to work. The edge of the internal condom hangs outside the body, so it covers more skin than a regular condom. You can use them in vaginas and anuses. If you're a penis-owner who has difficulty using traditional condoms, internal condoms may be your salvation.

Dental dams are thin pieces of latex or nitrile that act as a barrier for cunnilingus or analingus. To use one, lay it flat against your partner's vulva or anus so it covers the whole area, hold it in place, and go to town. If you don't know how to use a dental dam, you're not alone. Dental dam use isn't common, but that doesn't mean you shouldn't know how to use one just in case.

Gloves are great for hand sex. They protect against long or sharp fingernails, hold lube better, and cover any small cuts you might have. They also make safer sex easier because you can touch yourself with the same hand by removing or replacing the glove. They come in lots of colors to avoid that "dentist" look.

PRO TIP

Some people in monogamous or closed relationships often choose no barriers. This can be done safely if you're both STI-free and don't have sex with other people. Others who choose to have sex without barriers may do so by getting tested regularly and having conversations with their partners about their status. If you have P/V sex, though, you're still going to have to figure out contraception (see page 199).

Bottom line: you have options. Some folks choose to play it super safe by using barriers for everything and not kissing. Others may choose to use barriers only for penetrative sex, or decide on protocols based on the relationship they have with each partner. The most important thing is *you* choose your protocols.

As with any boundary, if your partner refuses to compromise or figure out a win-win that makes you feel safe and appreciated, I suggest reevaluating whether that's a good person to be intimate with at all.

Personally, I have a hormonal IUD and have barrier-less sex with my cis-male primary partner. I use condoms for all other P/V sex and barriers for oral sex if requested. I like to use gloves for hand sex, though sometimes I'll go without. I'm happy to accommodate safer sex requests and I always have a safer sex conversation before we get to the sexin'. I get tested every six months.

HANDLING POSITIVES

Okay, so you got tested and something came back positive. Now what? Odds are, some sort of emotion will come up. You may feel gross or scared or resentful. Feel your feelings and take care not to lash out at yourself or others. Once you've processed your feelings, enlist your logical brain to help calm down your freak-out response. The fact is, most STIs are curable, treatable, and not that big of a deal. Chlamydia, gonorrhea, syphilis, and trichomoniasis are all treatable and are often easier to manage than a cold. Herpes can be treated with medication that can reduce or eliminate breakouts. HIV is manageable with daily medication and is far less terrifying than it was even ten years ago. HPV can be managed with medication and surgical procedures. Yes, these can be complicated by other health issues, but that's no different than any other communicable disease.

The clinic that delivers the positive result will likely offer you treatment right away. But sometimes your doctor may recommend a "wait and see" approach (as is common with abnormal Paps that may or may not indicate HPV). As soon as you get your results, share them with your partners so they can get tested as well. Read on to the STI Disclosure section below for a good way to communicate the news.

Everyone relates to STIs differently. Some of us are pretty chill on the whole and don't freak out when we learn we've been exposed. Others can take it really hard, for both logical and less-logical reasons. It's not your job to control other people's emotions. Give them the information they need to take proactive steps to take care of their own bodies and let them process their emotions.

Even if you're a germaphobe or hypochondriac, you don't have to let fear of STIs keep you from enjoying a sex life. Many clinics and doctors will let you set up a regular biannual or quarterly testing schedule. Have safer sex conversations well before sexy-time so you can mentally prepare for any issues. Get vaccinated. Create safer sex protocols that make you feel safe during sex. Research the stuff that scares you. The reality is almost always less frightening than the stories you've heard. This is especially true if the sex ed you got growing up was based on fear-mongering tactics and gross images of untreated diseases. Be proactive and realize you have more control than you might think.

STI DISCLOSURE

At what point should you disclose your STI status to another person? Good consent rules say as soon as *your* health becomes *their* issue. That is, as soon as whatever you have could be communicable to another person. Think of it this way: Have you ever met someone when you were sick? You may have said something like, "I'd shake your hand, but I have a cold, so I'd better not."

It's common courtesy to acknowledge you may be putting another person's health at risk by sharing contact with them. It's the same with STI status. If you tested positive, let your partners know. A good way to say it is "I *may* have exposed you to ____." The reason for this wording is you can't guarantee whether or not someone has been exposed to something, and you *definitely* can't tell for certain whether or not they've contracted it. We are all constantly exposed to a variety of things, from the flu to strep. That's part of being in society. Yes, it can be hard to have the conversation. If you need a model for how to do it, refer to ReidAboutSex's Difficult Conversation Formula over on page 105.

Disclosures are an opportunity to preserve trust and respect, raise everyone's sexual health IQ, and improve your community's sexual resilience. Here's the rub, though: You can't communicate your health status to someone *if you don't know what it is*. Get tested regularly. It's the only way to be sure you're sharing the right information (and not the wrong infections).

PRO TIP

Endeavor to use the word "clear" or "negative" instead of "clean" when discussing your status. People with STIs aren't "unclean" and we don't need to reinforce that kind of stigma.

Physical Safety versus Emotional Safety

Physical safety is straightforward: Preservation of your physical health and bodily integrity. Emotional safety can be more nebulous: Preservation of your emotional health and mental integrity. You can engage in play that's physically safe, but is emotionally edgy (cheating, for instance, or some kinds of kink). Similarly, you might feel emotionally safe but your physical safety is compromised if your partner has an undiagnosed STI.

Knowing the difference between physical and emotional safety is key to negotiating safer sex boundaries. If you don't know that one of your protocols is really an emotional safety thing, not a physical one, it can be hard to communicate with your partner(s) why you need something. The bottom line: Your boundaries are your own. You get to decide what makes you feel safe. It's your body, and it's your choice.

> Whenever my partner comes back from a long time on the road, I like to use condoms with him. It's not that his travel sex is any more or less risky than usual. It's an emotional thing—before I can really drop back in with him and feel safe having unprotected P/V sex, I need to use a barrier a few times. Once we figured out that I had an emotional safety need, and it wasn't stemming from a lack of trust, it became part of our reconnection ritual.

Emotional insecurity often stems from wobbly communication and incomplete information. So get the information you need, whatever it is. Reread this chapter, get tested, drill down on your anxieties, and figure out your protocols.

Then, practice talking about this stuff. Share your protocols with your friends, and ask them to share theirs. Get this conversation so well handled that it doesn't feel scary or complicated, but just another thing to discuss.

Vet potential sex partners on their ability to show up for the conversation. Are they squicked out? Slut-shamey? Enthusiastic? Nervous but open? Their response will give you a TON of information about their emotional maturity and how well they handle their safer sex needs. No single response has to be a deal breaker, but it's all helpful for vetting.

You can alleviate many of your sex life woes simply by upgrading whom you sleep with, and you will know how to upgrade those people when you see how well they respond to your sharing. If you scare a potential sexy-time prospect away by initiating a conversation on safer sex needs, that just means they're not playing at your level. You want to be knockin' boots with the awesome people who are taking their own sexual health into account (and yours by extension).

Contraception

We're blessed to live in a time where there are a lot of options for birth control (BC). My general rule regarding contraception: Protect yourself. Take responsibility for your own fertility, regardless of your gender, and take precautions to prevent creating an unwanted pregnancy. There are three main forms of birth control: hormonal, mechanical, and surgical.

Hormonal birth control alters the body's systems to prevent pregnancy in ways such as thickening cervical mucus to prevent sperm from entering the uterus or stopping ovaries from releasing eggs at all, so there's nothing to fertilize. Here are some examples of hormonal birth control:

→ **The Patch.** A plastic sticker that releases hormones. Applied weekly.

→ **The Ring.** A rubbery, hormone-containing ring worn inside the vagina. Kept in for three weeks or can be used continuously to prevent periods.

→ **Birth control shot.** Hormonal shot that lasts three months.

→ **Subdermal implant.** A tiny metal rod implanted under the skin of your arm that will release hormones for up to four years.

→ **Birth control pill.** Daily hormone pill. Can be taken continuously to prevent menstruation.

→ **Hormonal intrauterine device (IUD).** A small, plastic, T-shaped device containing progestin that is placed inside the uterus to prevent fertilized eggs from implanting; lasts 3 to 6 years. Copper IUDs are made of metal and don't include hormones, but they function similarly to hormonal IUDs.

→ **Long-term sex hormone use.** Some trans people can reduce their fertility with prolonged hormone use. Trans women on androgen inhibitors often have reduced sperm counts and trans men on testosterone often stop ovulating. Everyone is different, though, and your particular dosage may impact your production of sex cells. So it's a good idea to use some sort of protection in addition to hormones to avoid pregnancy. On the flip side, some trans folks can reduce their usual hormone intake if they want to try for pregnancy. The effectiveness of this strategy varies. If you're not sure if you want to make a baby in the future, before beginning hormonal treatments, consider freezing your sperm/egg cells for future use.

PROS: Often make menstrual cycles lighter and shorter. Some hormonal methods may stop menstruation completely. Depending on the kind you use, it can last for a day, a month, a few months, or years. Usually really effective. Many don't require daily thought and can allow for more "spontaneous" sex. Don't affect sexual sensations.

CONS: None of these prevent STIs, just pregnancy. Some folks just don't like messing with their natural hormones. Can require a doctor's visit, a prescription, or other ongoing expenses. Can have negative interactions with other medication or cigarettes. Efficacy relies on consistent use/exposure. Negative side effects can include mood swings, heavy cramping, or irregular periods. For IUDs, implants, or shots, you won't be able to get pregnant until you remove the device and/or the hormones wear off.

> After years of considering it, I finally got an IUD (Mirena). My period stopped, my PMS is negligible, and I feel safer having P/V sex in general. In short, I fucking love it. Insertion was rough, though. The standard pain-relief recommendation for IUD insertion is a couple of ibuprofen, but I knew that a li'l headache pill was not going to cut it. I asked my doctor for some heavier drugs and she prescribed me an anti-anxiety pill, a muscle relaxant, and a heavy-duty painkiller. Insertion still sucked, but it sucked just that much less. If you're like me, talk to your doctor about your options. When it comes time to get my IUD replaced, you bet I'll be asking for a similar cocktail.

If you're on the fence, you can try hormonal BC for a few months and then decide if you like it or not. (The removal of IUDs and implants can suck, but it's better than living with something you don't want in your body.)

Emergency contraception (EC) is hormonal birth control used on a case-by-case post-facto basis.

→ **The Morning-after pill/Plan B.** Essentially a megadose of Levonorgestrel, the active ingredient in birth control pills. It prevents ovulation, and if ovulation already happened, it prevents the egg from implanting on the uterine wall. Available over the counter at pharmacies or online, and there's no age limit in the United States. Can be taken up to five days after unprotected sex, though it's best taken within three days. If you're a regular sex-haver, it's a good idea to have some EC on hand for emergencies, and let your friends know you have some too in case they need it. The shelf-life for EC is a few years. There's some controversy as to whether EC has a weight limit. Research has shown Plan B has a reduced efficacy in people over 175 pounds. Some EC manufacturers suggest folks over 175 take two of the pills instead of one.

→ **Ella/Ulipristal.** Ella is another brand of morning-after pill that has a different chemical makeup that makes it more effective than Plan B after three days and more effective for people over 175 pounds. Currently, Ella is only available in the United States with a prescription.

→ **Super emergency contraceptive.** Should you not be able to access Plan B but *can* access normal birth control pills, taking four to five at a time approximates the effect of Plan B. This is what's known as the "Yuzpe Method."

→ **The abortion pill.** Formerly known as RU-486, this pill is a safe, effective way to end a pregnancy up to seventy days after your first missed period.

PROS: Can be used after the fact to prevent or terminate a pregnancy. Generally safe. One time use rather than ongoing. Can be used as back-up if a mechanical BC method fails.

CONS: EC can cause nausea, cramping, depression, fatigue, migraine, and all the other things you might associate with a brutal period. Must be taken in a timely fashion to work. Some forms require a prescription. In many states, administration of the abortion pill requires clinical supervision.

Mechanical birth control is a physical barrier that prevents sperm from accessing the egg. Here are some mechanical birth control options:

→ **Condoms.** Thin latex or nitrile sheaths that either cover the penis (external condoms) or are placed inside the vagina (internal condoms), preventing ejaculate from entering the uterus. Disposable.

→ **Diaphragm.** A reusable silicone cup that covers the cervix.

→ **Cervical cap.** A reusable plastic cap that covers the cervix and contains spermicide.

→ **The sponge.** A disposable piece of foam that contains spermicide.

PROS: They're just used for sex, so there are no hormones changing your natural cycles. They're affordable and most don't affect the way sex feels at all. Some of them (like the sponge, diaphragm, and cap) can be inserted/applied hours before sex starts so you can still feel "spontaneous."

CONS: Some people don't react well to spermicide. If you use these methods incorrectly, pregnancy is definitely possible. They need to be inserted at most a few hours before sex, so unlike hormonal BC there are no "set it and forget it" options. You need to have them on hand, so if you're out of your preferred contraception you may be out of luck. Again, only condoms prevent STI transmission.

Surgical birth control is altering your pipes to prevent eggs and sperm from ever meeting IRL. Some options include:

→ **Tubal ligation (sterilization).** A permanent surgical procedure that stops ovulation by cutting or sealing the fallopian tubes. Many doctors won't perform this procedure if you've never had kids or can't prove you never, ever want them. This is both infuriating and patronizing, but it's true. So you may need to doctor-shop a bit before you find a physician willing to listen to you. Sometimes insurance covers it, but not always.

→ **Vasectomy.** A simple outpatient surgery in which the vas deferens (the tubes that carry sperm to the urethra) are cut and sutured, preventing sperm from entering the ejaculate. Vasectomies are 99 percent effective, reversible multiple times, and don't affect sexual performance, pleasure, ejaculate volume, or hormone levels. In the United States, most health insurance covers all or part of the cost of a vasectomy, and it's one of the best things you can do to protect everyone from unwanted pregnancy.

→ **Hysterectomy and Orchiectomy.** Some people elect to have some or all of their reproductive organs surgically removed completely. These procedures are generally performed on people with chronic issues related to these organs or folks who can "prove" to their doctor they are trans. Both hysterectomy (uterus removal) and orchiectomy (testicle removal) have significant hormonal implications, so find a doctor (usually one who is trans-friendly) to discuss these options.

In addition to vasectomy and condom use, here are a few things penis-owners can do to help mitigate pregnancy risk.

→ **Ejaculation control.** For many penis-owners, ejaculation can often feel inevitable and impossible to control. But with intention and practice, ejaculation control can be learned. It's a useful sex skill that will allow you to prolong the pleasure for everyone involved. It also allows you to decide *where* to come, which can offer practical and erotic opportunities. If you're interested in developing the skill, check out Taoist and Neo-Tantra sex and meditation practices. However, using ejaculation control as your *only* birth control is a bad idea. Sperm can be present in precum and even experts can lose control every once in a while. Add another form of BC to protect yourselves.

→ **Checking the condom.** Get in the habit of making sure the condom is still in place and intact before coming. Though they're reliable when applied correctly, condoms can still sometimes slip or tear. This is yet one more reason to develop ejaculation control, so you can double check everything looks good before letting 'er rip.

For more thorough explanation of all your birth control options, visit PlannedParenthood.org/learn. While you're there, make a donation. Planned

Parenthood is a wonderful, life-saving organization that can use all the help it can get to keep educating people about safe sex.

The bottom line to all this: Handle your shit. If there's a mistake, own it and take steps to mitigate the consequences. Don't just cross your fingers and hope for the best. Find your preferred contraception method and use it. Have EC on hand for emergencies. Sleep with people who handle *their* shit, and who respect your body and your choices.

Abortion

The best way to avoid having to get an abortion is by not needing one in the first place. If you do need one, here's what to know:

→ Abortion is legal in the United States. Some states are working hard at making that not true. Federally, the fact is, abortion is legal.

→ Abortion is safe. Safer than a colonoscopy. Safer than a tonsillectomy. And *much* safer than carrying a pregnancy to term.[1]

→ Abortion is health care.

→ Abortion is a human right.

→ Even though they can cost $$$, abortions are cheaper than carrying a pregnancy to term. Some health insurance covers abortion.

→ More than two-thirds of abortions happen in the first trimester. It's often cheaper and easier to manage in the first trimester, too. If you think you could be pregnant, take a test ASAP (after your first missed period, or starting a week after unprotected sex).

→ Roughly one-third of abortions performed in the United States are medication abortions (aka the Abortion Pill).[2] These abortions are non-invasive and can be completed at home. The rest are surgical proce-dures that require a clinic visit.

PRO TIP

Crisis pregnancy centers (CPCs) are scams run by forced-birth activists who try to scare people into carrying unwanted pregnancies to term. Be extra careful when using your Maps app to find an abortion provider, because CPCs try to game the system to trick people into thinking they provide resources that they don't. If you need to find an abortion clinic or want to know more about your options, contact Plannedparenthood.org instead.

SUPPORTING SOMEONE THROUGH ABORTION

If a friend or lover needs an abortion, you can help financially, emotionally, and/or practically. Take to the internet and help research. Many clinics use gender-normative language (i.e., referring to all abortion-seekers as women, etc.) which may be alienating for nonbinary and transmasculine people. If necessary, contact clinics about their policy for nonbinary/transmasculinity identities.

If you're partially responsible for the pregnancy, helping pay for the procedure is a decent thing to do. If you weren't involved, but you have the means, you can still offer to pitch in. (And consider donating to Abortionfunds.org to help other people who don't have awesome friends like you.)

Both surgical and medical abortions can make it hard to drive home afterward and, depending on the state, clinics can be far and few between. If a road trip is warranted, you can help by offering to drive.

Remember that everyone relates to abortions differently. Some folks may be super chill about it. Others may need to mourn or process. Don't expect your friend to behave in any sort of "right" way. Just offer your support and love as needed.

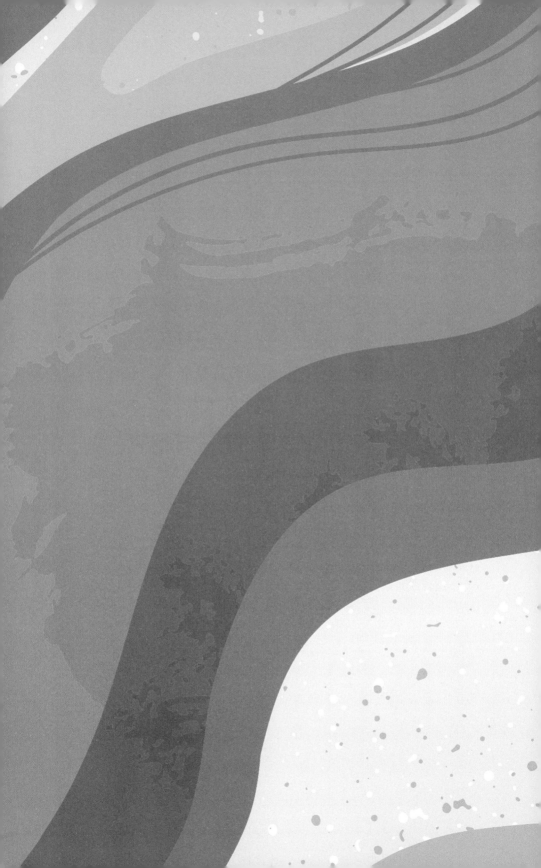

Heads, Hearts, and Other Parts

For some, sharing your body is the ultimate act of vulnerability. For others, it's sharing your heart. Either way, intimacy is a practice. It's a commitment to the belief that we are stronger and sexier when we walk toward vulnerability, openness, and grace. True, sex doesn't have to be intimate. It can be perfunctory or businesslike. But it can be extra rewarding when we choose partners who can hold space for vulnerability, and offer some of their own as well.

Radical Vulnerability

I'm guessing you know what it's like to hold your tongue. You probably know how to pretend you're not feeling something you are very much feeling. You might not be able to describe it, but if you could, you might say it feels like a tightness in your chest or throat, or your shoulders bunch up, or you want to cry but can't. You might feel like you have words you can't utter, or you're achy or wounded in a nonspecific way.

I'd be willing to bet not only do you know what it feels like, but most of us experience it in some form every day. Our culture shames loneliness, sadness, and yearning. It mocks genuine expressions of love and pain. So we shut it down, tune it out, and go on pretending we don't feel anything at all.

Sex is all about vulnerability. We bare our bodies and expose our most delicate parts to one another. We worry about our performance, sounds we make, the way we touch, and the way we allow ourselves to be touched. We show each other parts of ourselves (physical, emotional, and intellectual) that we never show the rest of the world.

We try to deny the delicacy of this by trading emotional vulnerability for the physical sort. "If I'm going to let this person into my body," we seem to say, "I'll be damned if I let them into my heart, too." We can go full tilt into the opposite direction after casual sex, denying we felt anything beyond some transient physical pleasure. Any feelings we do have, we may shut down. Sure, we may probe the other person a bit, to see what's allowed. We'll wonder if it's "too much" to wake up next to them and have an intimate conversation over coffee. We'll try to divine their intentions and expectations, and try to align our emotions with what's reasonable. We ask for what we think we can get, rather than what we really want.

Society grants us different levels of vulnerability based on our identities. Vulnerability is a gendered thing. We permit it—almost expect it—from women and feminine types. We deny it—almost condemn it—from men and masculine types. We've come to describe this phenomenon as part of "toxic masculinity," wherein the most insidious aspects of what our society defines as "masculine" are pathologically prioritized and amplified, and otherwise benign or positive aspects of masculinity turn malignant. We exalt terseness and callousness. We prize stoicism and steadfastness. We idolize violence and aggression. We mock tears and tenderness. We equate softness with weakness.

These cultural narratives run deep. It can take a lifetime to learn how to be brave enough to face another person raw and openly. The tides are beginning to turn. We're starting to point to the problem and invite people to deconstruct their programming. We're starting to tell boys it's okay to cry and be frightened. We're starting to allow men to share platonic, tender affection with one another. Our granddads didn't have that privilege. In many subcultures, men and boys still don't have it.

Women and nonbinary folks often feel as if we have to play by these rules to be taken seriously, too. We pretend sex doesn't mean anything to us either, so we can keep on having it without being called "crazy" or "needy."

The result is we're all rounding our emotions down to their most blunt and meaningless expressions. We'd rather feel nothing than too much. We'd rather be seen as cold than desperate. We jump in and out of beds pretending none of it matters, when we're actually leaving the best damn part of sex in the hallway outside.

My advice: Let it matter. Aloofness is pointless. Being disaffected by sex is a mistake. Instead, we should strive to be *affected*. Let things in. Feel things. Have big, sweeping conversations. Witness one another. Be giddy and silly and bold.

Be brave enough to feel.

Being vulnerable doesn't mean info-dumping or using a one-night stand for free therapy. It simply means being brave enough to share what's on your mind when it comes up. It means not lying to yourself or your bed buddy about what's real for you. My hope is that we can collectively learn to open our hearts along with our bodies when we have sex. Not forever, necessarily—perhaps not even past the moment we put on our shoes to leave—but in that time that we connect, I'd like us to feel safe connecting fully and fearlessly.

When it comes to sex and relationships, I endeavor to be a beacon of permission, and let everyone know that things get better the more we're willing to be brave with our emotions. It may feel antithetical to remove the armor and the calluses to grow stronger, but it really does work that way. Try it. Next time you match with someone on a dating app or have lunch with a sweetie, try being radically vulnerable. Say something true you think will scare the other person off. Say something you think you can't possibly be loved for. If you do, and they stick around? Congratulations, you're having a real relationship.

So how do we step into vulnerability?

→ **Resist the urge to hide.** This is hard for many of us. Some of us are good at using sex to hide rather than reveal.

→ **Resist the urge to silence yourself.** There are plenty of logical reasons to silence yourself in life. Saying what's on your mind in a clear voice to ensure that you're heard is badass.

→ **Be willing to explore the range of experience.** You don't have to go full tilt into everything, but if you're curious about something, it's brave to try something you've never done before.

→ **Learn to become profoundly aware of your needs and desires.** In a society that expects us to subsume our passions, this is key.

→ **Allow yourself to be in a process of becoming.** Our society rewards certainty. It asks us to entrench ourselves in our identities and defend the boundaries of expectations. The truth is, there is no arrival, no destination. Life is just an ever-unfolding play of passion, despair, joy, and intimacy.

→ **Ask for what you want.** We're taught not to be too needy. Asking for what we want from another person is brave.

→ **Cop to your emotions.** You're allowed to feel things for the people you sleep with. In fact, I encourage it. Have your feelings, interrogate them when necessary, but otherwise let them be a part of who you are.

→ **Honor your word.** Say what you mean. Mean what you say. Back up your words with action.

→ **Admit when you fuck up.** Infallibility is impossible and absurd. Be brave enough to be fallible. If you hurt someone, fib, or deny your lived experience, admit it and take steps to heal the harm you caused.

These aren't just good ways to explore your sexuality, but good ways to go through life. Practice honoring the whole of your humanity and inviting other people to do the same with you. You may be surprised by how rewarding you may find it.

Look Ma, No Feelings!

Some folks think the best way to manage the complex emotions sex can arouse is by deadening their senses, either by using psychotropic substances or by disengaging with their emotions entirely. This is actually the opposite of a good idea. You know who don't have feelings? Psychopaths. You know who do have feelings? Decent people.

Instead of working hard to become dead inside, give yourself the opportunity to feel things before, during, and after sex. Sex can be an incredible teacher, but to learn you must be willing to feel. Sometimes those feelings lead to pain, so we try to nip them in the bud by tamping down our emotions. Any shrink worth their degree will tell you that denying emotions is a great way to make sure they stick around to torment you.

So rather than repressing your emotions, lean into the experience. It'll change so much.

Notice: As soon as you feel something, just notice you're feeling it. Acknowledge it with language if you can. Put a name to it.

> "I feel jealous."

> "I'm nauseous and I don't know why."

> "I'm feeling manic right now."

1   **Respect.** Once we notice we're having feelings, we might try to negate or rationalize them away. Acknowledge that feelings exist to direct our attention. Practice gratitude for your feelings, and allow them to tell you what they need to say.

2   **Engage.** Not all emotions need to be interrogated, and often it's a fine idea to feel your feelings as they come and let them pass. However, sometimes your emotions may make you feel out of control or unsafe. You may need to engage with your emotions to help guide them to a more healthy or compassionate place. Self-inquiry is a good place to start engaging with your emotions. After you've noticed what you're feeling and given yourself the opportunity to feel it, consider the source of the emotion. If you're feeling overwhelmed, begin your inquiry with

some grounding questions: "Am I physically safe right now?" "Am I able to take a few deep breaths?"

3   **Take action (maybe).** Sometimes your emotions point to actions you can take, like relationships to end or ambitions to pursue. If that is your situation, start engaging your logical brain to create a course of action. Other times your emotions merely need to be metabolized so you can go back to your life. Venting to friends is a good way to process, as is working stuff out with a therapist. You may choose to process emotions in the form of an artistic or athletic practice. Whatever it is, integrate this processing into your life so that when you know you have something big come up, you can tackle it proactively.

Love, Optional

Some people think of sex as a fun exchange of energy, and it shouldn't be any more tied to love than sharing a nice dinner, dancing, or connected conversation. Some believe romantic love should be a prerequisite to sex. Others don't think of love as a prereq, but that it makes the sex better. I have my opinions, and you'll have yours. For the moment, let's assume you want to have fun, fulfilling sex but avoid falling in love. Is it possible to share orgasms without sharing your heart? I think so, but it's not as easy as just willing it to be so. There's some neurohacking to try. Here are some guidelines:

Know yourself. Are you the kind of person who gets gaga over one kiss? Is oral sex the ultimate intimate act? Do you just love falling in love? Do you have an addictive personality? Love highs are real. Know yourself and choose accordingly. You just might not have a personality that can handle sluttery.

Find your people. If after every romp your friends ask, "Are they the one?!" that's going to put a lot of pressure on you. Hang out with people who get it.

Sleep with those people. If after orgasm your sex partner asks, "Am I the one?!" you're doing it wrong. If you want to sleep around, but you're doing it with people who want monogamy, *you're* the jerk. Sleep with other people who get it.

Public/group sex helps. Orgies, play parties, and sex clubs are great ways to have a good time without getting into the one-on-one habit.

Once (a month) is enough. If you only see each other once or twice a month, and you only see each other for sex (as opposed to date-like things), you can help avoid the oxytocin spiral. Just remember **KISSS: K**eep **I**t **S**eldom and **S**imple, **S**lut.

Diversify. If you're relying on one person to meet all your emotional and physical needs, you're in the danger zone. Diversify your community, and source your needs from multiple people. That may mean you have a cuddle buddy, a movie buddy, a go-out-dancing buddy, a bath-time buddy, a BDSM buddy, and a couple fuck buddies. This helps you reduce the hormonal hit you get from one person and spreads out the yummy feelings of connection and love over multiple people.

Are We . . . Dating?

Sometimes when you're hooking up with the same person over and over, you can experience a bit of "mission creep." That is, you start out as NSA fuck buddies, then you're FWBs, and then you're sleeping over all the time, and before you know it . . .

"Are we . . . dating?"

If you find yourself wondering what you are to someone else, the best way to figure it out is to open up a dialogue. It's normal to be nervous. It can feel vulnerable to have feelings you aren't sure are reciprocated. There are three routes you can take:

1   **Scale it back.** Take it back to basics. Consider adding rules to keep the mission creep from creeping back in. Maybe no more sleepovers, or only getting together for sex and no social time. Whatever makes you feel like you're back on an even footing.

2   **Roll with it and see how it develops.** This means answering the "Are we dating?" question with ". . . I guess so?" If that feels right for both of you, great!

3   **Cold-turkey it for a while and see what feelings arise.** This is like pushing the reset button on your relationship. If you're missing

the sex and not much more, that's a sign all you need is to get laid and you and your buddy are particularly compatible. If you find yourself pining after the *person*, well, maybe you did develop romantic-type feelings after all. Decide how to proceed from there.

Falling in Love

Uh oh. You fooled around and fell in love.

It happens to the best of us.

So . . . what now?

Well, you have some options. You can share your feelings and ask to take the relationship to the next level. You can work through your emotions on your own and keep your sexy friend in blissful ignorance. Then there's the nuclear option: shut it down, fake your death, move to a new city, and change your name. Each has their pros and cons, but let's not go nuclear just yet.

> Penelope was supposed to be a fling. We'd fooled around here and there, but it felt like a mutual crush and little more. When she came to town for work, I was giddy to see her. I had plans that evening and gave her a choice of sleeping arrangements. When I came home late at night, I found her in my bed. I tried to slip into the room quietly, but she stirred. "Did I wake you?" I asked. "No, I waited up," she replied. That night we had intense, romantic sex. As the weekend progressed, it was clear we were both smitten. When I dropped her off at the airport, an obvious question hung in the air: "When can I see you again?" The unspoken answer was, "As soon as we can manage."

Know that love, like lust, is chemical. It's a neurological process like anything else. Your glands are squeezing hormones into your bloodstream that make R&B songs play in your head whenever you see their face. Your neurons are firing in a "Yes, please! Nom good!" pattern whenever you get a whiff of their scent. Your gonads are screaming "Baby-making! Yes, please!" whenever you rub up against them.

Welcome to meat-sack sentience.

So, knowing you may be acting and feeling a wee bit irrational as your brain does the conga through your heart to your genitals and back, how do you deal?

First, acknowledge your feelings, even if they scare the living shit out of you. Denying your feelings never quenches them. So let 'em flow like The Force through the Love Jedi that is you. Admit it. You're smitten. It feels giddy and fun and you may as well enjoy it because it doesn't happen every day.

Then, give it a logical once-over. Did this person just rock your world in the sack? Are they the only source of non-mechanized orgasms in your life? Note that. It may merely be lust or relief disguised as the real deal. If, however, the feels are deeper and more resonant, then yeah, you may be sliding headlong into love.

But ask yourself, "Do I actually *want* to date my fuck buddy? Are they boy/boi/girl/gurl/squish/squash-friend material?" Take some time with this one, because the answer may be hard to suss out. I've had hot and heavy crushes that made me gaga, but when I stepped away and thought, "Do I want to be this person's girlfriend?" the answer was a shocking and resounding "Fuck no!"

If it's a "Fuck yes," offer an opt-in. Let them know, but don't coerce. Some folks try to maneuver their fuck buddies into being romantic. They may try to make the sex more connected or trick them into going on dates or whatever. That's not nice. If you're wanting to take things from fuck buddy to love interest, have the conversation.

If they're on the same page, you'll probably experience a fun cocktail of relief and terror. Ain't it grand? If they aren't on the same page, continuing your sexual relationship may bring endless heartache. It may be best to take some time off to reassess or end the relationship completely. I'm not going to pretend this is easy. In fact, it SUCKS. But sometimes taking time and space is what your heart needs to find a way through. Create distance if necessary, and let your sweetie know what you're doing and why. Give it some time and step back in. If you have a good thing, it'll still be there in six months.

New Relationship Energy

New Relationship Energy (NRE) is a term coined in the polyamory world for describing that gaga feeling you get when you start seeing a new, shiny person. Some folks get NRE all the time, whereas others get it for certain people that hit them right in the hormones. Either way, it's a good idea to know what to expect so you don't (1) feel insane and (2) annoy the shit out of your friends and lovers.

NRE can be one of the best parts of dating. You feel giddy, silly, awkward, love-drunk, and high. In fact, feeling high is an accurate description for it. Neuroscience shows that when you fall in love, you experience a cascade of neurological effects akin to being addicted to cocaine. Since it's applicable, let's borrow some advice from addiction experts:

→ **Admit you have a problem.** You are high. Your drug is Your Person. Acknowledge it's a neurological issue and your rational brain has little control.

→ **Place your trust in a higher power.** I'm an atheist, so the higher power I choose to defer to is Time. You might choose Sanity or Brain Chemistry or the Muses or whatever.

→ **Trust time to take the edge off.** Ride it out, and you'll almost always end up in a better, more serene place where you can be more rational and composed.

→ **Figure out if there's something else off in your life.** Feeling empty or directionless? Perhaps a little codependent? Investigate yourself to see if there's something you need to improve to avoid allowing NRE to clobber you and diving into gaga land.

→ **Maintain a balanced life.** Resist the urge to make rash life decisions and merge your identity and life with this new person. It's common to want to blow up your life and start fresh when you fall for someone new. You might decide to drop everything, quit your job, and travel across the world to be with your person. My advice: *don't*. Give it at least six months, though nine is better. If the urge to go AWOL is still there after nine months, you might consider it real. Anything less and you're likely making decisions with your genitals, not your mind.

→ **Support your lovers and peers through their own NRE stuff.** Call them out if you see them being dickish. Stand up for yourself if you're feeling harmed or neglected. Help raise the emotional resiliency of your entire community.

PRO TIP

It's easy to neglect other partners and lovers when you're really into a new person. Once the NRE wears off, though, you may find you've also worn out the sweeties you've been ignoring. Try to honor your agreements and be attentive to everyone's needs, even when you're batshit over a new person.

Hey, Jealousy

Jealousy happens. The problem is many of us were raised to avoid jealousy at all costs. This means when it does come for us, it tends to clobber us like an ogre. Meanwhile, others are taught that jealousy is how we *prove* love, and behaving in ways that inspire jealousy in our lovers or demonstrate our own jealous rage are a good thing. Either way, we are often unequipped to handle jealousy. So while we may have good tools to survive other emotions, jealousy can take us out at the knees. But just like sadness and lust are responses to a combination of internal and external forces, so is jealousy. It usually strikes when something's off about how you're feeling with yourself and how things are going in your life.

Like with any feeling, the first thing to do is notice it. There's no shame or weakness in being jealous. It's a normal part of being alive, and it doesn't make you "less evolved" than your friends. That said, realize **your jealousy is your responsibility.** Yes, it's possible someone did something to elicit the emotional response in you, but it's still your emotion. So own it. You are allowed to ask your partner(s) for support, but just like they shouldn't be expected to fix your life when you feel sad, it's also not their job to make the jealousy go away. That's on you. Shore up your own reserves first, *then* ask for support.

Figure out what's off. Are you feeling lonely? Abandoned? Broke? Undesirable? Think back to what was happening right before jealousy hit you, and determine the stimulus, understanding it could be a combination of factors.

My partner Reid Mihalko and his colleague Dr. Beth identified eight main jealousy triggers in what he calls the "Eight-Armed Octopus of Jealousy." Here are the beast's "tentacles":

- → Loneliness
- → Need to feel special
- → Fairness/equity
- → Loss/fear of abandonment
- → Rejection
- → Insecurity (in the relationship)
- → Inferiority (feeling "less than" within one's self)
- → Longing/scarcity

Sometimes having one tentacle get tugged is enough to set you off. For other folks, it takes two or three tentacles getting pulled to trigger a jealousy attack. Take a look at the list and figure out which ones are your likely triggers, then figure out ways to neutralize them. Lonely? Schedule a friend date. Insecure in the relationship? Ask for reassurance. Feeling scarcity? Make plans with your sweetie that you can look forward to.

Think of jealousy like the check engine light on your car dashboard. That light doesn't mean you're a bad driver. It doesn't mean pull over right away and call 911. It doesn't mean you should sell your car and commit to never driving again. It's just an indicator that something needs to be addressed. Your car is telling you, "Hey, this is a thing you should look at so I work well and stay healthy." So it is with jealousy. Once you notice what's up, you have the power to intervene before shit gets wonky. That check engine light might be telling you that you need more quality time with lovers, or you need to attend to things that bring you joy, or you need to focus on a spiritual practice, or whatever. If you give it attention and thought, you'll figure it out.

> While it's great to make requests or ask for reassurance, respect your partner's other relationships. It's rude to demand your partner's attention when they're on a date with someone else. Work through your shit on your own, then have the conversation when they're available.

A cool thing about getting good at handling jealousy is now when I feel jealous, I'm grateful. Not maybe at the moment, because yeah, it still totally sucks. But when I get jealous, I know to investigate what's going on in my life. Sometimes it's as simple as I need a nap. Other times it can indicate I need to take a hard look at my life and my choices. Whatever it is, jealousy is a sign pointing to something that needs fixing in your life.

IT'S NOT ME, IT'S YOU

If you're fooling around with different people, you may find yourself dealing with a jealous lover. Here's the most important thing to know: There's a difference between bad feelings and abuse. An indicator is how much they use *their* feelings to try to control *your* actions. For instance, jealousy is "I'm feeling sad you're going out with your friends tonight. Can we make a date for tomorrow?" Abuse is "I'm feeling sad you're going out with your friends tonight, so I'm going to be mean to you until you 'offer' to cancel." If your partner slut-shames you, threatens you, or otherwise makes you feel unsafe because they're jealous, that's a big ol' neon sign flashing "Abuse." If your lover uses their jealousy to manipulate you, shame you, or invade your privacy, that's not okay. Draw your boundaries and get support.

Healthy relationships involve compromise on both ends. Abusive relationships tend to be more unilateral. Your sweetie may have been taught that jealousy was a way of showing love. But real love is about respect, not control. Bad feelings happen, but they shouldn't derail a respectful, compassionate relationship. If they do, that's a sign that your relationship may not be healthy.

Assuming you're dealing with the more benign "I love you but I feel crappy" kind of jealousy, begin with compassion. Your partner isn't a bad person or stupid just for feeling jealous. Avoid shaming your sweetie for having these feelings. If you aren't causing harm, it's not your job to fix anything. Sometimes people wield jealousy like a weapon to try to get you to behave the way they want you to. You are not obligated to allay their jealousy. That's *their* job.

That said, you can offer to brainstorm solutions. Sometimes people express feelings just to feel seen, and they don't want you to fix anything. If they *do* want your help, ask, **"How can I support you in getting your needs met?"** Offer affirmation, support, or whatever you feel comfortable contributing to the health of the relationship. For instance, you might suggest they call up friends they haven't seen in a while or take themselves out to a thing you wouldn't want to do with them anyway.

One of the most common causes of jealousy in casual sex situations is when one person is monogamous and/or falling in love and doesn't want to admit it. Trying to be chill when you're experiencing strong emotions can make you feel possessive. If you want your casual sex buddy to be your main squeeze, it's best to be honest rather than try to weasel the other lovers out of their life.

Even if your situation is casual, make an effort to give the relationship attention. Keep your word, make time for your connection, and show up for difficult conversations. Make sure everyone feels good about the state of the union.

After the initial hit of jealousy has faded, conduct an inquiry. Is everyone getting their needs met? Is everyone feeling respected, honored, and appreciated? That might feel like overkill for a fuck-buddy relationship, but if the fuck-buddyship is healthy, odds are, neither of you will doubt that you feel appreciated.

Codependence

Codependence is a common and commonly misunderstood phenomenon. It originated as a concept in alcohol treatment programs, but it has since evolved into a much more nuanced and far-reaching idea. Codependence often manifests as an addiction to an emotional state or relationship. It's often a way to deny the full integrity of your selfhood and subsume your identity into something external. Codependents often stake their emotional health and self-worth on their partner's emotional state. They may take blame for their partners' bad behaviors and go to extraordinary lengths to win their approval. They will often try to predict how their partner will react to something and will alter their behaviors to steer toward preferred outcomes. If you're afraid to ask for what you want, assert boundaries, or take pride in your own accomplishments (rather than exclusively on your partner's), you may be codependent.

If you suspect you have codependent tendencies, it doesn't mean you can't enjoy a healthy, diverse sex life. It just means you may need to be extra vigilant about maintaining your boundaries and honoring your own needs and identity. There are whole books dedicated to the subject (see page 270) and even twelve-step groups specifically for codependents (visit CoDA.org).

Attachment Styles

Attachment theory is a psychological concept that describes interpersonal relationship dynamics through different attachment styles. Originally developed to explore children's relationships with their parents, the model can also describe romantic and sexual relationships. How well a person feels attached to another often indicates how capable they feel exploring, taking risks, and trusting one another.

People who are **securely attached** favor direct communication, intimacy, and transparency in relationships. They feel safe being themselves, talking about their feelings, and honoring their partner's needs for intimacy.

People with **anxious-preoccupied attachment** can be hypervigilant, attempting to psychically divine what's going on in their partner's head. They often worry about doing or saying the wrong thing. If your favorite phrase is "Are you mad at me?" you may have an anxious attachment style.

Dismissive-avoidant attachment types tend to cut and run. They distrust others and are unreliable, especially when things get hard. These types can be workaholics or have a strong need to source self-confidence from their accomplishments rather than their relationships.

Fearful-avoidant folks have a more push-and-pull relationship with intimacy. They may want closeness, but fear they don't deserve it. They can be incredibly sensitive to even mild rejection and have a hard time asserting or maintaining boundaries. They may have low self-esteem, which may cause them to isolate.

Any of these styles can manifest in a relationship, and some of them are particularly relevant for people who have casual sex. If you're an avoidant type, for instance, it's much easier to move on to the next sex partner than to stick it out through a challenging but rewarding relationship moment.

Attachment styles can be conditional, too. You may generally be a securely attached person, but you meet someone who pushes all your anxiety buttons and you find yourself getting worked up in new (or more likely, *deeply familiar but forgotten*) ways. Your attachment style affects how you date, how you have sex, and how you break up. If you want to understand yourself and your partners better, diving into attachment theory is a great idea.

TRAUMA BONDING

Trauma bonding can occur when a partner is inconsistent with offering affection. Similar to codependency, trauma bonding can encourage people to try to predict their lover's mental state to elicit the "reward" of affection and avoid the punishment of denial or cruelty. People who are traumatically bonded hyper-analyze and control their behaviors to try to win their partner's fickle affection. The result is that people in a traumatic bond often feel confused, gaslit, and a little bit nuts.

Ever had amazing sex, then get ghosted, then have that sweetie drop into your DMs months later like nothing happened? Ever think you connected with someone, then they treat you like shit, then they gaslight you into thinking you have intimacy problems, then they say they want to "get serious"? If you feel a little out of control, trying to figure out how to make them happy and keep them crushing on you, even when they act erratically, you may be experiencing a trauma bond.

Recognize it, and discuss it. If there's a reason behind the inconsistency, figure it out. Ask for upgrades and consistency. It may be that your sweetie and you just aren't on the same page. But if it's because they have an avoidant or fearful attachment style, it's best to figure that out early and set some boundaries to spare your sanity.

Designing Your Relationships

Our society comes with lots of defaults for relationships and sex: heterosexuality, monogamy, vanilla sex, strict gender norms, marriage-and-kids, etc. We're lucky to be living through a time where these defaults are being deconstructed and revealed for the weak sauce that they are, but that doesn't mean we still don't fall victim to their sometimes insidious nature.

Even if we think we're being deliberate about designing our relationships, defaults can sneak in and lead us to make erroneous assumptions: We sleep with someone once and assume we're dating, we slip into unexamined gender roles regardless of whether they feel right for us, or we kink-shame our partner when we're confronted with a desire we find "too out there." When people don't want the same things we do, we can use the defaults against them to pathologize their preferences, labeling them as wrong or deviant. The good news is, when you're engaging in conscious, transparent casual sex, you're fighting against the defaults and helping others understand their real options. Do everyone a favor and talk through this stuff first:

Ask for their intentions and share your own. Talk to your partners about what they're looking for. If they're looking for love and you're looking for a roll in the hay, it doesn't have to be a deal breaker, but it does allow you both to make a more informed decision.

Fluid until proven otherwise. It's a good idea to invert the paradigm and assume no one wants monogamy until they say so. Same goes for the rest of the defaults. Try assuming no one is totally straight/gay, no one wants marriage and kids, no one is purely vanilla, and no one behaves like the platonic gender ideal until it's discussed. This helps you maintain a flexible mind and not get thrown by any new information.

Appreciate a good fit. A monogamous and polyamorous person can date. So can a queer person and a straight person or a kinky person and a vanilla person. You don't need complete parity in all things, just a good match for what you're looking for at that point in your life.

Honor transience. One of the beautiful things about casual sex is its impermanence. It forces us to appreciate the moment and enjoy what's right in front of us instead of what's to come.

Depth, Not Duration

One of the most powerful things we can do as romantic partners is adjust our metric as to what counts as "success" in relationships. Western culture's obsession with tenacity and stick-to-it-iveness means we tend to prize miserable long-term relationships over extraordinary short-term ones. We call divorces "failed marriages" regardless of how much love and appreciation were built and still remain.

Venerating duration is a result of transactional relationships. Just a few generations ago, marriage was mostly a business arrangement. It was a way to merge resources and create a safety net for aging family members. Love was a bonus, but not at all required. Tenacity was a virtue because your family's literal survival relied on your ability to "tough it out."

Now we have far more freedom to choose, and that choice may mean enjoying short-term relationships in lieu of long-term ones. If you want to upgrade your love life and explore more opportunities to connect, I suggest prizing depth over duration. Consider how well you can treat someone rather than how long you can stand them.

I'm sitting at the dining table in my New York pied-à-terre. My lover Scott has just left for the day, and I'm sipping the last of the iced coffee he ran to the corner to buy while I was waking up.

Despite the giddy fun of a new love affair, there's a bittersweetness to it. See, Scott is monogamous. He wants (one) wife and kids. I'm polyamorous, in a committed primary partnership, and I never want to be a parent. There is a time limit on our relationship, and it will likely end as soon as Scott falls in love with his next partner.

Sure, I could decide not to be with Scott to spare my future self some pain. Or I could appreciate him now, knowing my life will have been richer with him in it, even when we transition away from sex.

I've had romances like this in the past—amazing humans who wanted different things than I did, but we made sure to appreciate each other while the moment was right. There's a wistfulness to these relationships, a built-in ephemera.

> These relationships, where you go deep and love well, knowing a whistle will eventually blow and the game will be over, can be some of the most enriching and healing intimate relationships one can have with another person.

You don't have to hide behind the artifice of "future" with partners. You don't have to weave fantasies or create a solid foundation upon which to build long-term love. When you prize depth over duration, you get to meet each other where you are, share what you're about, and enjoy.

Nonmonogamy

Nonmonogamy is a feature, not a bug, of casual sex. The assumption with casual sex is that everyone is a free agent and can sleep with whomever else they want. So you may be practicing nonmonogamy even if you didn't think you were the type.

A great benefit of ethical nonmonogamy (e.g., polyamory, swinging, relationship anarchy, etc.) is not having to forsake your other lovers when you start seeing anyone more intensely. You can still take things to the next level with one or more people, while maintaining stasis with your other sweeties.

My favorite thing about being nonmonogamous is being free to take every relationship on its own terms. I don't have to temper my feelings or my desires to keep my partners feeling safe. In fact, me being self-expressed is precisely what makes them feel safe, knowing I can have sex with and date whomever, but none of that will make me leave them. Likewise, I want to know about my partners' feelings. I want to know who they love and how. That, to me, is real intimacy. So all my partners know all about the other ones, and it makes me feel extra loved and safe to know everyone is on the same page.

* * *

If you suspect you'd want to keep your sexy friends as sexy friends even if some of those friends become more, you might be a nonmonogamous person to the core. You have options when it comes to what kind of ethical open relationship might work for you.

→ **Swinging:** Hetero couple-based, for the most part. Sexually open but romance/love relationships are usually not part of the deal.

→ **Polyamory:** Sexual and romantic openness. Boundaries and rules are negotiated to work for everyone involved on a case-by-case basis.

→ **Closed polyfidelity:** Romantic configurations of three or more people who are in a "closed" relationship, i.e., they don't see other people outside of their arrangement. You may hear terms such as "closed quad" or "closed V" to describe these situations.

→ **Sex work:** Some folks may be monogamous unless it's for work.

→ **Relationship anarchy:** Everyone is a free agent and no one has to answer to anyone about how they share their bodies or hearts.

→ **Monogam-ish:** A *mostly* monogamous relationship, with the ability to play outside every once in a while (either as a couple or solo).

If you suspect your desire for sexual openness is more than just a slut phase, lead with it. If you're not interested in monogamy, say so. It'll help you find other people who are in the same boat and can mitigate awkward relationship conversations down the road.

That said, keep in mind that nonmonogamy isn't a panacea. Many people have tried nonmonogamy and totally fucked it up. If you aren't great at asking for what you want and asserting boundaries, openness won't fix that. Luckily, we live in an age where more people are out about their nonmonogamous lifestyles. Use their knowledge to avoid some of the more common pitfalls.

Some folks are ardent that relationship orientation is just as intrinsic to one's identity as their sexual orientation. I can see that, but I also think that life is complex and fascinating. There are indeed people who choose their relationship orientation, just as there are people who choose their sexual orientation. You may go through a phase where you're monogamous and then decide to be nonmonogamous. You may date a partner who wants monogamy, so you opt in, even if it's not your preference. Choose your choice, and honor the agreements that go with it. Be willing to reevaluate that choice every so often to make sure you're still contented and fulfilled.

FUCKING WHILE MONOGAMOUS

Casual sex doesn't belong to the nonmonogamous. It's a viable choice for people regardless of their relationship orientation and sexual appetites. Everyone is entitled to a slut phase. Sometimes that phase is your twenties, sometimes it's after a divorce, and sometimes it's your whole life. Even if you're searching for that one special someone to settle down with, you can have fun, casual romps on your way to finding that person. The first thing to consider is: Are you really monogamous? Monogamy is such a default in our society, few people ever give themselves a chance to wonder what kind of relationship they actually want.

Remember the Ideal Sex Life exercise way back on page 16? Try it again, this time envisioning your ideal *love* relationship. Just the two of you until death do you part? Sexual monogamy but deep, intimate friendships? Checking out a sex party with your spouse every once in a while? Certain sex acts okay with other people? Something else? Remember, there are innumerable ways to structure a relationship, so give yourself some time to think about your ideal fit.

Once you have a sense of what you want your future to be, think about the present. Even if you're monogamous, you may want different things from your slut phase. Some folks may want to date and sleep around as way of finding The One. There are plenty of long-term relationships that began as one-night stands. Other folks may want to sleep around between relationships as a way of dealing with heartbreak or learning about themselves before they start seeking a capital-R Relationship. You may want to figure out some stuff or just get it out of your system before you commit to monogamy.

Regardless of the why, figure it out so you can discuss it with dates. You'll likely meet other monogamous people in their own slut phase, and you can decide if your versions are compatible.

Hiring Pros

Hiring a sex worker (SW) can be a great way to explore sexuality with built-in boundaries. Sex workers can help you practice initiating/negotiating sex, or help you get more comfortable with people's bodies (or your own!).

Depending on where you live, it's possible (or likely) many kinds of sex work are illegal. Government raids of databases and provider sites have made it harder to find professionals, and they've made those professionals much choosier in how they advertise and connect with clients. I recommend finding individual sex workers you like on social media sites, like Twitter, then asking how they book clients. Sometimes they'll have booking info right in their profiles. It's also okay to ask for referrals if you're looking for a specific thing the SW you're talking to may not provide. If you're not sure who you're looking for, try some of the larger searchable databases such as Slixa.com.

Sex work is like any other profession: there are specialists and generalists. Take some time to consider what you want from the exchange. Explore a specific fetish? Test your boundaries and learn more about yourself? Learn a skill? Experience intimate touch in a safe space? The more specific and open you are about your interests, the better the professional will be able to meet your needs.

Expect to jump through some hoops when booking. Some sex workers establish rigorous protocols to protect themselves from time-wasters, cops, and creeps. Don't complain or ask to skip the line. The sex worker is vetting you based on your willingness and ability to play by their rules.

Remember back in the slut-shaming chapter when I said people who get slut-shamed the worst are those who are societally disadvantaged? Well, sex workers are it, bud. This is why most police procedural TV shows are built around Dead Hookers™. Sex workers are so thoroughly slut-shamed in our culture that we don't even treat them as fully human, and we're okay with them "getting what they deserve" as a cheap plot device. Banks, social media, Hollywood, and, of course the Feds have it out for them. So be *extra good* to sex workers. They deserve respect, appreciation, and cold hard cash for all the nonsense they put up with.

Remember, this is a business relationship. The sex worker probably won't offer personal details, and they don't want to be your sweetie. Think of it as a body worker relationship. Yes, they're going to touch you, and yes, you're going to feel things. And yes, they have their own personal life that doesn't involve you. They're doing their job, and you're paying them for it.

So act gentlemanly (even if you're a lady). Treat the sex worker with respect and dignity. Don't ask for freebies. Don't be rude or dismissive (outside of a negotiated scene). Don't expect them to relax their boundaries for you.

If you care about a sexually healthy society, it's a good idea to care about sex workers' rights. Signal-boost activist movements, donate to sex worker causes (like Red Umbrella Project and Sex Workers Outreach Project), and speak out about decriminalization.

I am unabashedly and unreservedly pro sex work. Learning how to get into the business is outside the purview of this book, however. If you enjoy sex enough to want to turn it into a side or full-time hustle, check out the Recommended Reading section (page 270).

The Business
of Breaking
Hearts

There may come a time when you have to end things. There's no guarantee how it'll go, especially when hearts and egos are on the line. On the easy end of things, you'll say, "Hey this isn't working out for me" and they'll say, "Yeah, me neither. Take care," and you'll both walk away feeling satisfied. I've had those kinds of breakups before; they're a little magical each time. On the other end of the spectrum, there are breakups where the neighbors call the cops. As a general life rule: the fewer cops, the better.

PRO TIP

The depth and length of the relationship isn't directly related to how easy the breakup will be. I've had easy breakups after six years of being in love, and complete garbage breakups after six months of texting and a couple romps. There are no guarantees when it comes to sex and love.

First, do some solo work:

Name what's not working. Get clear with yourself about what's making you unhappy or uninvested in the relationship. Do you feel underappreciated? Are they not satisfying your sexual needs? Do you want something that the other person isn't willing to give? Or vice versa? It can be shallow or deep, doesn't matter. Just name it.

Examine your list of grievances. Decide which ones are deal breakers and which are workable. If the list is all workable things, would it be better to try to improve the relationship together?

Do a gut check. When you contemplate your relationship, how do you feel? What does your gut tell you about whether or not you want to try to work it out?

* * *

Once you've decided you want to break the news, aim for doing it face-to-face. A phone call is the next best thing. Avoid text messages or emails, unless you the need the safety of distance.

Be timely. Don't drag your feet. Make time for the conversation.

Focus on "I . . ." statements. Only speak on behalf of your own needs or desires that aren't being fulfilled by the relationship.

"I'm ready to meet someone who wants kids, too."

"Long distance has made it hard for me to focus. I need to date people in my city."

"I'm starting to fall in love with you and if you're not available for that, I need to step back."

If you're coming up with blaming or "you" statements, take some time to reframe first. For example:

"You never prioritize me" → "I need someone who puts me first."

"You only want sex" → "I'm looking for a more well-rounded and emotionally fulfilling relationship."

"Your drug use is a problem" → "I need to spend more time in sober environments."

Own your shit. If things went sideways, take responsibility for what contribution you made to that dynamic. This can mean apologizing, demonstrating what you've learned, and maybe seeking out professional help if it looks like a chronic issue.

Be compassionate. Don't coddle or infantilize the person, but do treat them with care. This shit is hard. Don't fear their emotions. If you're breaking someone's heart, have the patience and decency to hold space for them without judgment or minimizing. Also, be kind to your own emotions as well. Emotional vulnerability can feel far more frightening than physical vulnerability. For many of us, it's easier to say, "Fuck me harder, Daddy!" than, "I think I'm falling in love with you."

Be honest. Don't lie about why you're breaking it off and don't keep them on the hook just because it feels nicer than making it final.

Be thorough. It may be tempting to omit key details to spare feelings (like if, say, you've fallen for someone else). However, this creates ambiguity that can feed confusion and bargaining. So, if you decided you want to be monogamous with someone or you've lost the spark or you're just not happy with the arrangement anymore, say so.

Be grateful. Thank them for being a good friend/fuck buddy/lover for the time you were together. Say something you appreciated about your time together:

> "Spending time with you helped heal my heart after my big breakup."

> "Thank you for introducing me to [insert kink you now enjoy]."

> "I had a lot of fun with you both in and out of bed. Thanks for being rad."

Be clear on next steps. Are you taking a little break? Or is this a final decision? You might be surprised at how many broken hearts come from one person holding out hope of retrying in the future, when the other one is sure it's over. Don't say you'll revisit things in six months if you don't mean it. If you *feel* final about your decision, *be* final about it.

If your breakup buddy needs another conversation after the first one, consider granting them that generosity. It's important to have some time to digest new information. Sometimes it takes a couple breakup conversations for it to stick.

Don't ghost. Stopping returning texts and calls is so childish and shitty; it infuriates me just thinking about it. Be a grown-up and talk to the person. You're role modeling to them how to be in future relationships, improving the emotional skills of your whole community.

Allow room for their emotions, but don't tolerate abuse. We all handle rejection differently. It can kick up sadness, anger, frustration, and confusion. There's nothing wrong with feelings. However, when someone can't handle rejection, they may get abusive. If this happens, draw a boundary and leave the situation. You can let them know you're open to talking again once they've cooled down, if you're up for that.

If you decide to continue some sort of relationship/friendship, show up for it. Sometimes you're lovers or you're nothing. But other times, you may want to continue to have them in your life. Most of my closest friendships are with former lovers. There's a beautiful kind of friendship that can blossom from sexual relationships. If you want that, take extra care with each other during the breakup to make sure there's enough respect and trust to build a foundation for a solid friendship.

> Last year I got dumped twice in three weeks. The first was utter garbage. We didn't discuss our feelings or thoughts or needs, we just knew something was borked. I spent months after trying to figure out what the fuck had happened.
>
> The second breakup was a fucking dream, I shit you not. Penelope called me up and explained her feelings, what she needed from her life, how our long-distance situation was having a deleterious effect on her mental health, and what kind of relationship she hoped we could build together in the future. She was so kind, thoughtful, and thorough that if I didn't let her dump me, *I* would have been the asshole. After an hour on the phone, I loved, and appreciated her more than ever before.

Show up for the conversation, and be willing to try a few times to get it right. No need to harp or dwell, but hopefully you'll get to a point of clarity where you address the imbalance and right it, or end it.

Welcome to the Lonely Hearts Club

The amount of heartbreak felt after being dumped is *not* proportional to the length or seriousness of your relationship. In fact, you may be caught off guard by how deeply you'll hurt after the breakup of a "casual" situation.

It's okay to be sad. Heartbreak is a nearly universal experience that causes real emotional and physical pain. It's common to experience depression, anxiety, sleep disorders, digestion issues, and sometimes even PTSD from heartache. So give yourself permission to be a mess for a little while.

If your ex-sweetie wants to hang out like nothing's wrong, you're allowed to let them know you're not ready. Acting cool and disaffected is a losing strategy. Be honest with them, with your friends, and, most important, *yourself* about what you're feeling.

Feed your soul. Surround yourself with friends. Do things for your body, heart, and mind that nurture you. But above all, give it time. There are a million songs about how time heals all wounds. In the case of heartbreak, it just happens to be true. You may need to take a few weeks or months to mend, but when you're ready to stop dwelling, I *strongly* encourage you to get back out there and flirt with some folks. Breakups can rattle your sense of self-worth. So give yourself the chance to feel fuckable again. It'll really help.

> I never expected to start a relationship with Scott. When we met, I was hung up on a different guy entirely, and Scott was going through a brutal breakup. I had a spare theater ticket the "other guy" was supposed to use, so I invited Scott out as a friend. When he showed up, I was surprised by my attraction to him. I asked him if he'd like to fool around, to distract each other from our heartache. That night, we found solace in one another. I felt chosen and desired. He felt appreciated and lovable. After our first night together, our relationship blossomed into a lovely FWB situation. We explored sexuality together, we healed hurt parts of ourselves, and we reminded one another we're sexy, loved, and appreciated.

The bottom line: This shit can suck for a while. That's part of the gig. If heartache lingers too long, if you get obsessive, abuse substances, isolate, or experience other major life disruptions, it's a good idea to seek some help.

WHAT NEXT?

After a split, some people need to go heal alone, while others need to stay in contact. Usually, this difference is based on how you process. There are two main types of processing: internal and external.

Internal processors need to take time alone to move through their feelings and come to conclusions. They tend to mull before having conversations. If you're an internal processor, you may want to go on a solo self-care trip, dive into creative projects, or practice mindfulness exercises, like yoga or meditation.

External processors prefer to talk through their feelings. They often need to stay connected through conflict, and process aloud. If you're an external processor, you may want to start seeing a therapist or make some friend-dates for support and venting.

Use your understanding of your processing style to make requests of your partner and make a plan for how to deal with the emotional fallout. Try to be explicit about your needs so they know why you're trying to stay connected or take some distance.

Once the initial breakup pain has passed, you may wonder if it's possible to go from lovers to friends. The short answer: sure! It's not always easy, particularly if the emotional investment was skewed toward one side in the relationship, but it's possible.

Figure out what you want and create an opt-in. If your ex will never be able to give you what you want, it may be better to sever ties. However, if you find that actually, you still enjoy going to concerts with your ex even if you don't sleep together afterward, you may find a new opportunity in your relationship.

It's easy to relax your standards when you're hurting, though. You might think, "Yeah, I prefer when my people stick to our plans, but I'll let my ex cancel on me twelve times because I miss them." Don't. Trust me. Lowering your standards so much that a geriatric snail could clear the hurdle into your heart is a recipe for resentment. Don't let someone make you feel terrible just because you'd rather have them nearby.

It's possible that new avenues of connection can open up between two people when sex is no longer the focal point. Consider your other options for connection and see what new things you can build together by appreciating what is. Our culture tends to prize romantic relationships above all others. Meanwhile, deep friendships can be some of the most fulfilling relationships in our lives. If you love sharing your time, heart, and intellect with someone, you may find it just as, if not more, fulfilling to continue the relationship, even if you don't share genitals anymore.

Josiah and I started as friends. Then we became friends with benefits, and before we knew it, we were in love. It looked a little different for both of us, though. Even at twenty-three, Josiah knew he wanted a wife and kids. He wanted me to move to London with him and get real. But I didn't want kids and wasn't the marrying type. I loved Josiah as an adventure buddy and lover. We both knew sooner or later we'd reach an unsolvable impasse or force an unfair compromise.

Despite our chemistry and happiness, we decided to dissolve our relationship so he could make room in his life for the woman he was looking for, and I could start my career in Los Angeles. True, at times it felt like I made a mistake, but because we ended it with love and respect, we got the treat of staying in each other's lives.

Six years after we broke up, I threw rice at his wedding, and two years after that, I bounced his first baby on my knee. No regrets.

The Tough Stuff

While I've spent time talking about how fun, expansive, and illuminating casual sex can be, the truth is, it's complicated business. Let's pay respect to the more complicated, painful, and intense things that sex can kick up.

Navigating Abuse

Here's a sobering statistic: One in four girls and one in six boys are sexually abused before they turn eighteen years old.[1]

So if you have sex with six people in your life, odds are at least one of them is a survivor of sexual abuse. Maybe you're a survivor, too. Abuse manifests in many different ways, and everyone heals at their own pace.

Some folks find casual sex to be part of the healing process. They may choose to remove some of the fear they have of other people by practicing being vulnerable with them. They may choose to take the power and mystery away from sex by mastering it. They may explore things such as kink and BDSM because they address complex issues such as control, humiliation, restraint, and pain in a more controlled environment.

If you're an abuse survivor interested in having sex as part of your healing process, make sure you're the one setting the pace and the terms. Find partners who will be patient with you. Sleep with people who are down for what you're down for. This doesn't mean they compromise their own boundaries, just that you both (or all) respect each others'. Even one-night stands can be considerate and flexible.

Also, explore soberly. Yes, alcohol and drugs can feel freeing. But they can also make it much harder for you to maintain control of a situation. So hew to activities and a pace that feels good when you're sober, even if that means moving slower than you'd hope to.

Explore different kinds of sex. Being adaptable and flexible are just good life skills, but they can be revolutionary when it comes to sex. There's so much more to sex than penis-penetrating-vagina. Experiment and find kinds of sex that feel good for everyone involved. Healing sexy touch can feel edgy, but it shouldn't feel like it pushes you *over* the edge.

Which also means, practice *self*-discovery. Though partnered sex can be revealing, it's equally—if not more—important to explore solo. Develop self-pleasure routines that involve touching yourself in healing ways. If there are parts of your body that are frightening for you to feel, it may be a good idea to develop a healthy relationship with them solo before inviting a partner's touch.

HOW TO BE A GOOD LOVER TO AN ABUSE SURVIVOR

Survivors can still have fun and hot sex. Still, it's good to be aware of how you can help make it safer for everyone:

Let them set the pace. Practice patience and compassion. Sometimes abuse survivors can act erratic or confusing. Sometimes everything will be swimming along until they shut down for some reason. Nothing is wrong, no one is broken. You just may have stumbled upon a trigger or memory. Pause and check in.

Negotiate up front. Talk about what you'd like, and encourage them to share, too. Many survivors have a difficult time speaking up. Talk about boundaries and hard limits before things start heating up.

Stay connected. Another common reaction to abuse is "checking out" or dissociating from one's body. If you notice your lover is suddenly not present with you (for example, not making eye contact, responding to questions, or reciprocating touch), pause and check in. Sometimes a simple yes or no question can do the trick, but other times you'll need to put everything on hold until you can reconnect.

Maintain your boundaries. Just because your lover is a survivor doesn't mean you have to give up your own sovereignty in service to them. You are entitled to your own boundaries. If they want to move faster than you do, you don't have to concede your desires to theirs. Be compassionate, but also advocate for yourself.

——————— **Panic and Fear** ———————

Sex can be intense. While that intensity often facilitates intimacy and arousal, sometimes it can kick up less-awesome feelings—like fear. Panic attacks happen. They can be hard when going about your daily life, but during sex, they can be devastating. You're not a bad or broken person if you have panic attacks. It just means your body is reacting to something outside your conscious control.

I was visiting my new lover, Alex. It was our second date, and our first sleepover. We were giddy. Things started well. We had chemistry. We were moving fast but we were both eager and sober. It was, in a word, *on*.

Twenty minutes after the clothes came off, we took our first interval. I was still nervous. I liked this guy. I *like* liked this guy.

Alex and I held each other and he told me in beautiful and specific words how much he liked me. Then he began to fall asleep. Anxiety gripped my spine. "Are you seriously falling asleep?" I asked. He rolled over and began to snore. I tried to speak, but my chest tightened and my lungs seized. I wanted to flee, tearing barefoot into the night, but first I needed to remember how to breathe. And anyway, my legs wouldn't work. I struggled to open my lungs, slow my pulse, and calm down.

I clutched my knees to my chest, tears welling at my eyes, for a painful fifteen minutes. Finally, my breath steadied and I came back to myself. I tried to curl up next to Alex, but he shook me off. So I lay in the fetal position, sleeping in fits and starts until sunrise.

A week later, I was at brunch with my ex, Naomi. I was still unsure what the hell happened. By this point, I'd told the story to a handful of friends. Each time, I ended the story with the punch line: "And then he fell asleep. Just like that." Women would gasp. Men would shake their heads. It was a funny anecdote. When I told the story to Naomi, though, she looked at me askance and asked, "Are you okay?"

I tried to laugh it off, but instead, I told the rest of the story. In the telling it became far clearer what had happened: I had a panic attack. As I spoke, I realized that Alex's falling asleep was a big trigger from an old abusive relationship. No one had ever triggered it before, so I had no idea it even existed.

My best advice is to treat trauma like asthma. Just like an asthmatic, you can learn to identify and avoid your triggers. Often a trigger has to get tripped before you know it's there, just like sometimes you have to pet a cat to realize you're allergic to cats. When it happens, notice it and add it to your catalog, without judging yourself. If you want to change the music, or the location, or whatever, there's no need to feel shame about it, just ask. If I were allergic to cats and my boo had a beloved feline, it wouldn't be unreasonable for me to ask them to come over to my place instead. Why should it be any different for trauma triggers?

Once you have a grasp of your triggers, practice exposure therapy—to the degree you want to, that is. If your trauma is centered around a certain kind of sex act, there's no rule that says you *must* learn to like that sex act. Fuck it. You don't have to do and like everything to be a sex-positive person. If you *do* want to learn how to appreciate something, however, take baby steps solo and/or with a trusted partner. The adage about anal sex works equally well for trauma: "the slower you go, the faster you get there."

When you find yourself in the middle of an attack, focus on breathing and acknowledge it's happening as soon as you can. This can help turn on your logical brain, which is your secret weapon during a panic attack. If you're with someone, naming it can help them understand what's happening. Try to ground yourself in the physical world. If you need to be held, ask to be held. Walking on grass or submerging your hands in warm water can help, too. Connect to your surroundings (by, say, counting all the blue objects in a room) to remind yourself you're not in immediate danger.

When you calm down, try to remember what it felt like as the panic attack approached. This can help you navigate when it happens the next time. The key to panic attacks is often turn-around time. You can't control when they happen, but you can learn how to put both hands back on the wheel. It gets easier with practice.

After that first panic attack, I had a few more, months apart. The second time it happened, I noticed the familiar feeling in my chest that said, "Run!" Luckily this time I was at a campout. So I ran into the woods and hugged a tree until I calmed down. The third time it happened, I was at a restaurant in Times Square (less convenient for running to the woods). But I could see it coming from so far off that I was able to excuse myself, walk outside, find a quiet alcove, and practice breathing. Each time, I've gotten better at keeping one hand on the wheel and calming myself down.

Healing Sex

Many of us seek out sex because we're looking to heal something from our past: a toxic relationship, an abusive history, body shame, or religious trauma, to name a few. Sexual healing is a real thing, and it can pack a punch.

My dear friend Sex Nerd Sandra says, "We often seek out sexual partners who offer us reparative opportunities." If we don't get the healing we're looking for, however, our experience of the sex can feel unfulfilling or even empty. So if you're on the prowl for some heavy-duty sexual healing, it pays to be extra deliberate about your goals. Be upfront with your partner, be vigilant about maintaining your boundaries moving forward, and then focus your energies on making it count.

PRO TIP

It may be a good idea to hire a sex-positive (and potentially kink-aware, queer-capable) therapist or a trauma-informed sex worker to help you on your path. Find the right fit and diversify your healing.

Get an opt-in. Your sex partners may not need to know exactly why you're having sex with them. But if there are specific things you need to work out, consider getting their opt-in. For instance, if you want to explore a certain kind of touch that's edgy for you, let them know so that if things go sideways they don't blame themselves. This is equally important for rough sex as it is for more psychological sorts of play and intimacy.

Go extra slow. Sex can bring up big emotions. That's a feature, not a bug. But it can get overwhelming, particularly if you're trying to heal on some sort of timeline. Give yourself extra time to feel into things, back off if necessary, and reassess.

Maintain strict boundaries. If there are certain sex acts that are off the table for you, communicate those to your partner. If they can't honor that boundary, find a new sex partner, end of story. The last thing anyone needs from healing sex is *more* trauma.

Respect your partner. Remember that a sex partner opting in for healing sex is doing you a big favor. Sure, they may have a good time, too. But it can be quite a responsibility to hold space for someone else's healing. Don't overstep their boundaries, and practice good check-ins. Particularly if you're engaging with pain play, BDSM, or power-exchange, get explicit ahead of time about what you want to experience, and don't force them beyond that role.

Right after my in-bed panic attack, I got lost in grim feelings. I knew I needed to release some deep and primal sobs I couldn't conjure on my own. I went home to my partner and asked for rough sex. I told him, "I don't want you to stop, even if I start to look upset. I promise I'll safe-word out if I need to. Is that okay with you?" He fucked me until I was nearly hyperventilating from all the crying. Afterward, I felt serene and calm for the first time in weeks. I was able to release some of the grief I had been holding on to for twenty years. We cuddled, and I offered him reassurance that he didn't hurt me and everything was okay.

Healing follows its own timeline. If you go into it expecting to be able to check off all the boxes and determine, "Yep! All better!" you're in for some disappointment. Sometimes you need the dust to settle in your mind to understand how an experience changed you. Just as you can't expect to lift a dumbbell ten times and have a big ol' bicep, you can't expect one healthy romp or therapy session to fix you up for good. Give yourself the time to heal incrementally. Play the long game.

Therapy

At some points in this book, I've recommended you seek out therapy to help you work through stuff. While I think this is solid advice, I offer it with a *huge* caveat: Therapists are people. Duh, right? But it's important to keep in mind, because therapists can be susceptible to all the sex-shame the rest of us live with. Many therapists pathologize healthy sexual behavior because it doesn't fit into their idea of "normal." To put it plainly: some therapists are slut-shaming jerks. Run like hell from these people. They don't deserve your time or money. Find someone who honors who you are. To find an affirming therapist, try looking through the the American Association of Sexuality Educators, Counselors, and Therapists, AASECT.org/referral -directory, or National Coalition for Sexual Freedom, NCSfreedom.org. Some psych terms to pay attention to are "aware" and "competent." In psychology lingo, "-aware" (as in "kink-aware" or "LGBTQ+-aware") means the therapist has some training in these topics and/or is okay discussing them in a nonpathological way. For instance, a kink-aware therapist may be okay with you describing the kinky scene that triggered a fight with your partner.

"-Competent" or "-knowledgeable" means the therapist has done significant training in the topic and sees clients that represent that demographic. They may share that identity or have a personal history that makes them particularly adept at discussing the topic.

Therapist hunting can feel like dating: find some potential fits, schedule a first meeting, and chat. And just like dating, it's a good idea to find someone whose values gel with yours. You may have to wade through some duds before you find the right match, but doing the work to find the right fit may make all the difference.

Once I understood what happened in DC and where it came from, I knew I had some heavy shit to process. I was nervous. I had never been in therapy before. My life, particularly my sex life, is one some might consider "deviant." I was worried if I discussed my sexual history or the relationship that kicked all this old stuff up, the therapist would pathologize aspects of my life that I think are quite healthy.

On my therapy quest, I developed a phrase that served me well. Each time I met with someone new, I said, *"I'm queer, I'm nonmonogamous, and I'm kinky. And none of those are the problem."*

Some therapists were thrown by this. Some said, "I might need more information, but I can help." The therapist I chose to work with said, "Those identities are integral to my own community, and I'm happy to work with you, taking into account the importance and validity of those identities to who you are as a person."

It's possible the other therapists I interviewed could have supported me whether or not they shared my identities. But I'm happy I found someone who not only understood, but *related*.

Sex Addiction

Sex addiction has gotten a lot of attention recently. Celebrities check themselves into rehab for it, infomarketers try to sell us products to "cure" it, and pundits use sex addiction to explain a myriad of social ills.

The problem with sex addiction as a diagnosis is it's a huge, scary term that's used to label pretty much anyone with nonnormative sexual appetites or interests. (Never mind that "normal" is a moving target dependent on race, class, subculture, religion, appearance, etc.) Many therapists and doctors aren't trained in sexual health, and live with the same sexual shame and fucked-up society as the rest of us. Queer people, trans people, children with healthy sexual curiosities, sex workers, kinky people, and all sorts of other folks have long been labeled by society as "deviants" and given all forms of sexual addiction diagnoses. The least fortunate among our sexual forebears were jailed, killed, or forced to undergo horrific medical interventions such as lobotomy, shock therapy, and castration to try and "fix" their deviance. (World War II hero Alan Turing is a prominent example, but there are scores more.)

Sex addition diagnoses still lack nuance in today's society. If we can't agree on what healthy sexuality looks like, how can anyone know whether or not they fit into what's "normal"? To put it more bluntly: **It's not you who's broken, it's society that's fucked.**

However, we know compulsive, self-destructive behavior is *totally* a thing, and sometimes this takes the form of sex. So . . . does that mean sex addiction is real after all?

Eeeeehhhhhh. . . . Yes and no.

Let's break it down. There are three levels to repetitive behavior: habits, compulsions, and addictions.

Habits are simply things you are used to doing in a certain way. You can have the habit of brushing your teeth after every meal, having a beer after work, or masturbating before bed. Habits can be healthy or not, but generally speaking, you can alter a habit with simple readjustments.

Compulsions are things your brain feels you *must* do, even when they defy rationality. Things such as washing your hands for six minutes or opening a door three times before entering are recognizable forms of obsessive-compulsive disorder (OCD). Compulsions can also look like an urge to check Facebook even when you don't want to or a need to run three miles after you eat ice cream. Your conscious brain might be telling you to stop, but you are *compelled* to do the thing anyway. Folks may develop compulsions to help them deal with anxiety, but often these compulsions *increase* anxiety. For instance, if you feel a compulsion to check your favorite porn site at work, even when you know your boss is monitoring your internet use, what may have begun as a self-soothing habit may turn into a compulsive behavior with real-world consequences.

Addictions are usually defined as compulsions with deleterious real-world consequences. Traditionally, clinicians defined addiction as a physical dependence on a substance (e.g., heroin, tobacco, etc.). Recently, though, some experts have broadened the definition of addiction to include what they call behavioral addictions, aka non-substance-based attachments to things such as social media, gambling, porn, shopping, and video games. The line between compulsion and addiction is pretty murky. Neuroscientists try to focus on neural reward pathways and genetic predispositions, but science isn't immune to politics. The Diagnostic and Statistical Manual of Mental Disorders (DSM), which therapists use to classify disorders, is always changing in response to new understandings of human behavior (and it should be noted, the DSM governing body as repeatedly refrained from adding "sex addiction" as a diagnosis). If you're a nerd for this kind of stuff, there are great thinkers examining the theory and politics of diagnoses, psychiatry and "perversion."

Here are two things to consider regarding sexual compulsion:

> **Control.** How able are you to make decisions when presented with your drug of choice?

> **Consequences.** What are the real-world ramifications of giving in to your compulsions?

Evaluating these two aspects of behavior can help you assess whether or not something is a problem.

Sexual compulsion can look like a fixation on a sexual fantasy or sexual acts to the exclusion of other aspects of a person's life. The compulsion can be harmful or not. But, when a fixation starts to have *significant, real-world consequences*, like, for example, blowing one's savings on sex workers or engaging in high-risk behavior as a form of self-destruction, that may indeed be a problem. When a person has compulsive sex as a symptom of *a different, undiagnosed mental illness*, sex can be a problem.

When you lose the ability to alter or cease your compulsive behavior such that you experience significant, deleterious consequences, you may be dealing with a diagnosable disorder.

"Sex addiction" is a *nonclinical* label for harmful, entrenched compulsive behavior, much like gambling addiction or disordered eating. But just like binge eaters aren't just *really into food, man*, sex addiction usually isn't about the sex. It's almost always about an underlying issue that needs treatment, like depression, schizophrenia, and anxiety, i.e. things good mental health professionals can treat without piling on a bunch of anti-sex cultural baggage.

Sex addiction is such a contentious issue because our culture can't delineate between sexphobia and actual unhealthy behavior, and therapists can be guilty of upholding retrograde sexual standards. As with slut-shaming, we use the label of "sex addict" to bludgeon people who act in ways that make us uncomfortable. It may, for example, be easier to label your cheating ex a "sex addict" instead of admitting, hey, your relationship had a lot of problems. It may be easier to label yourself a porn addict rather than seeking treatment for your depression.

If you are hooking up so much that you are destroying your life for it, then by all means, seek treatment for impulse-control disorders. If, however, you're ashamed because your religious sister is praying for you all the time or you went down a rabbit hole of super intense pornography or you had sex with twelve people in one night and holy cow that's a lot . . . you're probably not a sex addict. You're just an intrepid sexual adventurer stuck in a stuck-up society. It's a drag, sure, but consider how miserable you'd be if you were on the other side of the battle.

Taking a Break

Just like some folks might go vegetarian for a summer or stop drinking to assess their relationship to booze, sometimes it can feel good to take some time away from sex. The word *celibate* is from the Latin that means "to be unmarried," and it originally referred to religious clerics. Nowadays it's been conflated with "abstinence" and the words are often used interchangeably. The difference is that "abstinent" is a generic term that just means to not do something, whereas "celibate" often refers to a thoughtful and intentional choice to be sexually abstinent for a higher purpose.

Some people choose celibacy because their pursuit of sex is taking up too much time and energy, or they want to reacquaint with solo touch or self-worth. It can be the right choice for those who want to practice controlling their sexual energy or to learn to listen to their authentic sexual expression. It may also be a way to readjust priorities, break bad sexual habits, or redirect energy into other parts of one's life. Celibacy doesn't look like one thing, though. There are a few options to consider:

→ **No partnered sex, but masturbation to orgasm is allowed.** This can be good for resetting your relationships with other people while maintaining the health and stress-relief benefits of orgasm.

→ **Playing with sexual energy is okay, but no orgasms.** This can be good if orgasm isn't gratifying for you, or if you want to practice raising sexual energy in your body without releasing it. Masturbation without orgasm is sometimes known as "edging." Edging is allowing oneself to get to the "edge" of orgasm, and then pulling back. This can be a useful practice for people who come too quickly or want to develop "orgasmic dexterity." Penis-owners who practice Tantra sometimes explore masturbation without ejaculatory release learn to "recycle" the orgasmic energy back into the body.

→ **No raising of sexual energy at all.** This kind of celibacy is often associated with religious or spiritual pursuits. When sexual urges come up, these types of celibates will often meditate, pray, exercise, dance, practice martial arts, or breathe through the feeling until it passes. They may also avoid things that would inspire sexual feelings, such as film/TV or going places where people are freely expressed.

Being celibate can be a great choice. It doesn't mean you have to cut out intimacy from your life altogether. You can still connect with people in emotionally and physically fulfilling ways through things such as cuddling, massage, partnered masturbation, partnered yoga, bathing together, or dancing.

BREAKING YOUR SEX FAST

If after trying celibacy for a while you decide you like it, there's no reason why you should stop. True, despite our culture's super screwy relationship with sex, many folks still find it odd if someone is full-tilt celibate without being highly religious. But if you don't think sex is for you, then by all means, don't have it. It's your body and your path.

If you prefer being celibate or find it intrinsically easy, it's possible you're on the asexual spectrum. **Asexuality** has different varieties. For example: demisexuals prefer to get down with someone after they form a strong emotional bond, whereas romantic asexuals may dig affection but don't want sex. If you'd like information about asexuality, visit Asexuality.org.

If you're ready to get back in the game after a stint of celibacy, it's often best to go slow. Just like reintroducing food to your body after a fast, your senses have likely recalibrated to your new way of living and will need some time to readjust. This can be a very sexy step. Often your nerves will be all the more sensitive to touch, and your sex hormones may be more intense than usual. Savor the moment.

Sex and Spirituality

I believe pleasure exists not just to encourage us to make babies but to remind us what we're on Earth for: to love and be loved. Even for a month, even for an hour, even for a moment. That's why we have bodies, nerves, and orgasms. That's why our hearts and flesh rejoice at the touch of someone who we'll only know for a few minutes. That's why we build communities beyond blood relations. Because sex and spirit are inextricably linked.

That's what I think. What about you?

"I am Jewish and my tradition teaches that sexual pleasure is healthy, good, and holy. I love thinking of myself as a Jewish slut!"

"I was raised Catholic and there was a lot of shame within religion due to the fact I was gay. When I became Buddhist there was more self-awareness taught, which made me feel more sexually empowered."

"Sex can be a spiritual experience. There's something about the primitiveness and primalness of it that makes it feel connected to nature.

"I've had spiritual energetic connections with partners before, but don't feel that sexual intimacy and connection is always necessarily spiritual."

If you feel conflict between your sexual desires and your religion, here are some ways to cope:

Research other religions. Not to convert, necessarily, but to explore the vast ways humans have integrated sexual pleasure into their spiritual lives. Many indigenous North American religions, for example, embrace gender and sexuality in more holistic and compassionate ways than colonizer religions. Similarly, different forms of polytheism around the world have deities that embody sexual pleasure.

Find community within your religion to talk to about these things. It may not be in real life, but perhaps on online forums where you may feel safer asking tough questions.

Separate yourself. Be willing to disentangle your own relationship with your higher power from the relationship you're told to have by your religious community. Explore where your heart is in alignment with the teachings, and investigate where your gut diverges from the party line.

Consider your religion in historical context. When many sacred texts were written, women were considered closer to property than human, concepts such as hetero/bi/homosexuality didn't exist as we understand them today, and there was an emphasis on reproduction for survival purposes. Times have changed. It's possible your religion hasn't.

Strengthen community ties in other ways. Sometimes leaving a faith can mean leaving your community. But you may be able to find ways to stay connected even if you're not at weekly worship. Let your family know your (possible) rejection of your faith isn't a rejection of them. Partake of the traditions that nurture your community and be deliberate about maintaining cherished bonds.

Sexual Citizenship and Integrity

Most sex is private, but the philosophy and politics of sex are worthy of public discourse. I believe among the many reasons issues such as reproductive health, sex work, sexual violence, and LGBTQ+ rights are so fraught in public discourse is because we have a hard time as a culture grappling with what's public and what's private. Many people feel awkward as hell having frank conversations about sex, making it nigh impossible to discuss how laws and morals affect the way we live our lives. It's essential we get better at this as a culture, so we can process the complexity of sex as adults and keep fighting for a more sexually just world.

Sexual citizenship requires us all to be responsible, not just for ourselves, but for our communities. But to do so, we must be willing to discuss sex with our friends and peers. Sex is not a silo, sealed off and removed from other aspects of our lives. The personal is the political. We must be able to discuss not only pleasure and love, but pain and conflict, in ways that uphold our values and align with our own sense of integrity.

Abuse in Communities

I don't need to tell you there are bad seeds out there. Some people use sex to hurt and manipulate people. What makes sexual manipulation so insidious is that some of these baddies use society's ambivalent relationship to sex to maintain a culture of silence and shame. When rape victims aren't believed, when sex workers should "expect" to be harmed because of their jobs, when people fear being fired or excommunicated or imprisoned or exiled for their sexual preferences, this creates a fertile stomping ground for bad-faith actors. I'm not talking just about mustache-twirling villains, though. I'm talking about the person who never takes responsibility for their messes, or uses BDSM irresponsibly, or spreads gossip because it makes them feel important.

Wrongdoers thrive in communities where there's already drama and gossip. It allows their bad behavior to join the din of other complaints and eye-rolls and be overlooked as just part of the deal. Because harm exists on a spectrum, each of us has a sense of what's over the line. In community, individuals will have different lines, creating confusion as to how to proceed when someone's causing strife.

Just as the best way to fight off an infection is with a healthy immune system, the best way to build immunity to the sloppy and ill-willed is by shoring up the strength of yourself and your community.

Community standards are important. Some spaces, like social justice movements or sex party communities, state their community standards in the form of venue rules, membership agreements, or manifests. It may be worth coming up with your own community standards before they're necessary.

Community standards aren't just to protect individual victims, but to maintain a culture of transparency. If there are clear, stated standards, victims are more likely to share openly. If there are ways for wrong-doers to repair the harm they caused, they may be more likely to stay engaged in an accountability process instead of skipping out of one community and into another.

Even in the absence of explicit community standards, you can take steps to protect yourself and your friends. Transparency is key here, too. Activist and writer Audre Lorde said, "Your silence will not protect you." Keeping shameful secrets presents an opportunity for people to use those secrets against you. This doesn't mean you have to be out about everything in your life. Just know there's power in transparency, and fewer dark secrets means less blackmail fodder. Try to take pride in the nuances of your sexual identity. Think about where you're hiding and where you could stand to step into the light a bit.

PRO TIP

There's a difference between living with shame and staying in the closet, though they can look quite similar. The closet is a tool, a strategy. It's a means to survive in unwelcoming or unsafe environments. You can be in the closet but also proud of who you are. Yes, you can still be threatened with outing, but intrinsic hatred, like shame, is far more harmful than extrinsic ones, like contextual closeting.

Maintain personal standards. Be willing to tell a party host, "I won't come if so-and-so is there," and call out shenanigans when you see them. Encourage wrong-doers to take responsibility for their actions. Gather facts, encourage people to speak up, and bring the information to people who have the power to affect change. Don't share other people's stories without permission, though. Instead, endeavor to create a space where people are safe to share their own stories. Sometimes this means talking to community leaders, party hosts, or just the people in that person's life.

Strive to be a person your friends and community can trust. Let people make mistakes and then fix them. Hold space for the complexity of humanity by refraining from shit-talking and hypocritical judgments. Admit your own fallibility. These small things may make you the safest person someone knows.

Remember, no one deserves to be on the receiving end of sexual violations—not prostitutes, not sluts, not porn stars, not even criminals. Don't perpetuate a culture that considers some people deserving of harm.

Don't spread gossip, but don't ignore your intuition, either. Does the person make you feel a little crazy, like you can't trust yourself? That your memory of events is flawed or your judgment is askew? Gaslighting is when a person tries to convince you what you know to be true is wrong. It's an insidious way of getting you to stop trusting your inner sense of judgment and place your trust in that person instead. If you feel like this is happening to you, it's helpful to keep track of what's up. This might mean journaling or finding a trusted friend to confide in. You may need an outside pair of eyes on the situation to help you assess what's true.

Pay attention to people's actions, not just their words. Do they support and care for people regardless of their status? Do they try to isolate people or stir up drama? Do they make you feel like garbage until they need something from you, then flatter you to death? Be wary of people who make you feel like trash most of the time and shiny every so often.

Be deliberate with your language and labels. Not all bad partners are predators or sociopaths. Our current cultural tendency to use hyperbolic language to describe a range of human behaviors has a *minimizing* effect on real harm. Remember, harm exists on a spectrum. Speak to facts, not rumors. Address behaviors, not personalities. We all have insecurities and flaws, and sometimes those flaws make a mess and cause harm. Your job as a good sexual citizen is not to fix others' bad behavior or make a terrible partner into a good one. Another person's healing is always their responsibility. You can opt in to helping, but only if it is within your boundaries. Remember to put on your oxygen mask before assisting anyone else.

SEXUAL INTEGRITY

The single best thing you can do for your sex life is choose partners and friends based on their integrity. This doesn't mean seeking perfection, but rather paying attention to how a person shows up for the hard stuff. If things go sideways or communication is off; if you hurt each others' feelings or say the wrong thing; if you want to share something real but are scared—is your partner going to rise to the occasion?

Endeavor to play at the highest level you can and encourage others to step up, too. It will make everything, from flirting to sex to love to partnership, far more rewarding.

Good sexual citizens acknowledge that sexual choices do not exist in a vacuum. The choices you make influence all aspects of your life and the lives of those around you. When you make sexual choices that are in alignment with your values and ethics, you act with integrity. Integrity has two dictionary definitions that are relevant to sex:

in·teg·ri·ty /inˈtegrədē/ noun

1 **Adherence to moral and ethical principles; soundness of moral character; honesty.**
   A person with sexual integrity:

   → Honors agreements

   → Speaks up when necessary

   → Respects their body and the bodies of their partner(s)

   → Comes clean when necessary

   → Does not perpetuate or tolerate abuse, hatred, or bigotry

→ Respects the privacy and autonomy of others

→ Acknowledges one's own boundaries may not be the same as another person's

→ Honors their identity, and the identities of their community members and partner(s)

→ Fights for justice and freedom for all

2 The state of being whole, entire, or undiminished.
A person with sexual integrity also:

→ Examines their own desires and proclivities

→ Investigates their fears, concerns, and hang-ups

→ Questions their assumptions, about others and themselves

→ Tends to their physical health, as well as their emotional and spiritual health

→ Seeks partnership and community with people with integrity

→ Considers their sexuality to be an intrinsic part of their humanity, and gives it the same respect and consideration as spirituality, intellect, and emotional well-being

Sex in Public

We are making progress toward a more sexually equitable world, but there's still plenty of work to do. You can help shift our culture toward the abundant, the expansive, the joyous, and the free. Here's how to start:

Be a beacon. Be the friend that people can come to with sex questions. The number-one reason I got into sex ed was because I grew up as "the sex talk kid." Even as a young person, I was fascinated by sex. Not just the clandestine nitty-gritty, but the way people thought about it and talked about it. All my life I've had conversations with my peers about their curiosities, challenges, and fears around sex. Many of my sex ed peers have similar origin stories. No matter where you are geographically or culturally, you can have conversations with people about sex. Listen with care, offer fact-based information when appropriate, and share your own thoughts with grace and respect.

Share your stories. Encourage your friends to share theirs, too. So much of what we perceive to be "abnormal" regarding sex is based on our culture of silence. We think our masochistic fantasies are weird and gross, and erectile dysfunction only happens to old dudes. We think it's not okay to watch porn or run home on our lunch break to rub one out. We wonder how many sex partners is "too many" and what kind of kink is "too out there." But if we talked about this stuff with trusted friends, we'd discover we're all far more "normal" than we may think.

Listen to public firsthand accounts. If you want to better understand trans rights or sex worker rights or abortion rights, listen to people who live those lives. Let people speak for themselves. There is no such thing as people who are "voiceless," just those who are silenced and ignored. Stop letting politicians and cops control the narrative. Be willing to have your mind changed by people's personal stories.

Stay curious. Not just about sexual politics, but racial equity, economic movements, and social justice. Sexual freedom intersects with our lives in complex and fascinating ways. Keep learning.

Demand accountability from your politicians. Power relies on complicity. Shitty politicians rely on people not voting or voicing their concerns. Shine a light on issues you care about by demanding elected officials address them in public forums.

Push back on myths. There is no shortage of sex education in the world. There is, however, a shortage of attention paid to the real deal. Educate yourself and call out bullshit when you hear it. Don't allow nonsense to proliferate. Use your voice to affect real, functional change in the world.

EPILOGUE

Like most sex educators, I'm constantly hearing people's sex stories. Often I'm the only person in the world they've told. The stories are always fascinating and sometimes horrifying. Most of the stories start with a lie—about what was normal, what was right, or what so-and-so told them about sex.

I'm thinking of Peter, the British nonagenarian who showed me the strap-on his favorite sex worker used with him when he visited her on leave during World War II. He never told his wife about it, but he told me. I'm thinking of Vex, who was bound and kidnapped at the behest of her parents in the middle of the night, thrown into a van, and driven off to a "conversion" camp to get the gay tortured out of her. There's Natasha, who suffered violent UTIs because her husband said he didn't like the smell of her vagina, so she douched with household cleaners and perfume. And there's June, who had her first orgasm at eighty-two years old, and wept in my arms lamenting all the time she'd lost. There are hundreds more. All these stories began with a lie, but they persist because we fear talking to one another about sex.

We must change the narrative, starting with our friends, our lovers, and our families.

The world is terrifying right now. Our enemies prize shame and silence, and they encourage us to be competitors rather than collaborators. We must combat these forces by fighting for transparency, intimacy, collaboration, and joy.

We must learn from our mistakes, heal harm, and tend to our wounds—both individual and collective. We must use our strength and privileges to fight for the right of everyone to live sexually expressed lives. We must have difficult conversations and be willing to work always toward equity and love. We must bear witness to one another, and allow each other to be raw and human and beautiful and seen.

Sex itself isn't revolutionary. It is, in fact, one of the most mundane forces in the world. But the way we do it has the power to change *everything*.

Advocate for yourself. Support your friends. Seek out truth. Quash shame and rumors. Build a life that makes you feel embodied, joyous, and vital. Share your heart and body with those who treat it with love and respect, and endeavor to do the same for those who share theirs with you. The world we can build together is worth it.

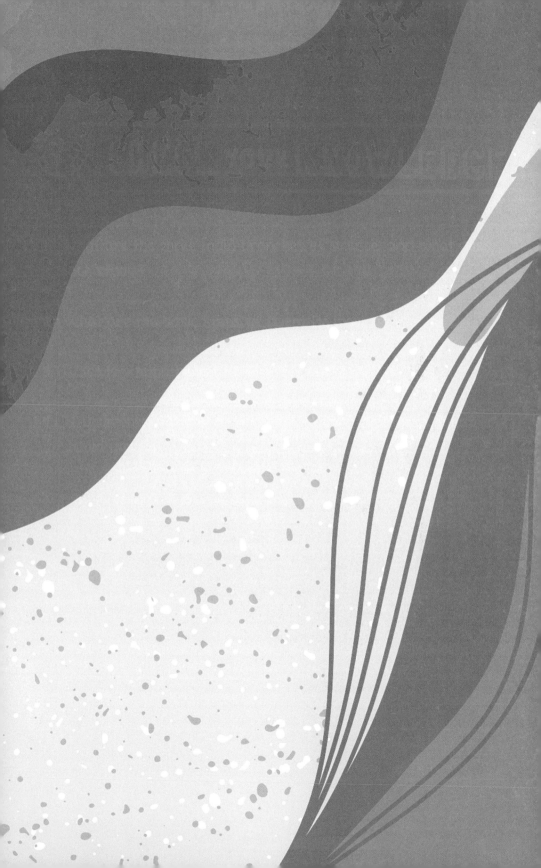

NOTES

Consent and Communication

BOOZE, WEED, AND OTHER DRUGS

1   Substance Abuse and Mental Health Services Administration Center for Substance Abuse Treatment, "A Provider's Introduction to Substance Abuse Treatment for Lesbian, Gay, Bisexual, and Transgender Individuals": https://store.samhsa.gov/system/files/sma12-4104.pdf

The Etiquette of Getting It

PARTNERED PLEASURE

1   https://link.springer.com/article/10.1007/s10508-017-0939-z

SEXUAL HEALTH

1   https://www.cdc.gov/hiv/basics/prep.html

2   https://www.cdc.gov/hpv/parents/vaccinesafety.html

3   https://www.ncbi.nlm.nih.gov/books/NBK47447

4   https://www.cdc.gov/std/trichomonas/stdfact-trichomoniasis.htm

CONTRACEPTION

1 https://journals.lww.com/greenjournal/Fulltext/2015/01000/
Incidence_of_Emergency_Department_Visits_and.29.aspx
https://www.thecut.com/2020/03/abortion-is-safer-than-getting
-your-wisdom-teeth out. html?utm_medium=s1&utm_
source=tw&utm_campaign=thecut

https://www.ncbi.nlm.nih.gov/pubmed/22270271

2 https://www.guttmacher.org/evidence-you-can-use/medication
-abortion?gclid=EAlaIQobChMI8vTut_2f6AIVBdVkCh02-wx8E
AAYAiAAEgLNFPD_BwE

Heads, Hearts, and Other Parts

THE TOUGH STUFF

1 Dube, S.R., Anda, R.F., Whitfield, C.L., et al. (2005). "Long-term consequences of childhood sexual abuse by gender of victim." *American
Journal of Preventive Medicine* 28, 430–438.

RECOMMENDED READING

SEXUAL EMPOWERMENT

Friedman, Jaclyn. *What You Really Really Want: The Smart Girl's Shame-Free Guide to Sex and Safety*. San Francisco: Seal Press, 2011.

Queen, Carol. *Exhibitionism for the Shy*. San Francisco: Down There Press, 2009.

CONSENT

Fischel, Joseph J. *Screw Consent: A Better Politics of Sexual Justice*. Oakland: University of California Press, 2019.

Martin, Betty. *The Wheel of Consent*, wheelofconsent.org.

TECHNIQUE

Carellas, Barbara. *Ecstasy Is Necessary: A Practical Guide*. Carlsbad, CA: Hay House, 2012

Chia, Mantak, and Douglas Abrams. *The Multi-Orgasmic Man: Sexual Secrets Every Man Should Know*. New York: HarperCollins, 1996.

Kerner, Ian. *She Comes First: The Thinking Man's Guide to Pleasuring a Woman*. New York: William Morrow, 2004.

Moon, Allison, and KD Diamond. *Girl Sex 101*. Lunatic Ink, 2018.

Nagoski, Emily. *Come As You Are: The Surprising New Science That Will Transform Your Sex Life*. New York: Simon & Schuster, 2015.

RELATIONSHIPS

Brown, Adrienne Renee. *Emergent Strategy: Shaping Change, Changing Worlds*. Chico, CA: AK Press, 2017.

Chen, Ching-In, Jai Dulani, and Leah Lakshmi Piepzna-Samarasinha. *The Revolution Starts at Home: Confronting Intimate Violence Within Activist Communities*. Chico, CA: AK Press, 2016.

Chapman, Gary, and Jennifer M. Thomas. *The Five Languages of Apology*. Chicago: Northfield Publishing, 2006.

de Becker, Gavin. *The Gift of Fear: And Other Survival Signals That Protect Us From Violence*. New York: Dell, 1998.

Donohue, Chris. *Sex Outside the Lines: Authentic Sexuality and a Sexually Dysfunctional Culture*. Dallas: Ben Bella Books, 2015.

Hardy, Janet W., and Dossie Easton. *The Ethical Slut: A Practical Guide to Polyamory, Open Relationships, and Other Freedoms in Sex and Love*. Emeryville, CA: Ten Speed Press, 2017.

Levine, Amir, and Rachel Heller. *Attached: The New Science of Adult Attachment and How It Can Help You Find—and Keep—Love*. New York: Tarcher, 2010.

Mellody, Pia. *Facing Codependence*. New York: Harper & Row, 2003.

Patterson, Kevin. *Love's Not Color Blind*. Portland, OR: Thorntree Press, 2018.

Richo, David. *How To Be An Adult in Relationships*. Boulder, CO: Shambala Publications, 2002.

Schulman, Sarah. *Conflict Is Not Abuse: Overstating Harm, Community Responsibility, and the Duty of Repair*. Vancouver, BC: Arsenal Pulp Press, 2017.

Van der Kolk, Bessel. *The Body Keeps the Score: Brain, Mind, and Body in the Healing of Trauma*. New York: Viking, 2014.

Zehr, Howard. *The Little Book of Restorative Justice*. New York: Good Books, 2015.

SEX WORK

Davina, Lola. *Thriving in Sex Work: Heartfelt Advice for Staying Sane in the Sex Industry: A Self-Help Book for Sex Workers*. Oakland, CA: Erotic as Power Press, 2018.

Lee, Jiz, ed. *Coming Out Like a Porn Star: Essays on Pornography, Protection, and Privacy*. Los Angeles: ThreeL Media, 2015.

Mac, Juno, and Molly Smith. *Revolting Prostitutes: The Fight for Sex Workers' Rights*. New York: Verso, 2018.

ACKNOWLEDGMENTS

Like good sex, this book was a collaboration.

Thank you to my agent Alyssa Jeanette at Stonesong Press for being enthusiastic about my perversity.

Thanks to Kimmy Tejasindhu and Kaitlin Ketchum for their insights and guidance. You have made this book better, and in doing so, have made me a better writer. To Annie Marino and the rest of the team at Ten Speed Press, thank you for making this book real.

To Rachel Keller, Luke Tracy, and Zita Zenda, thank you for letting me go a little feral in your guest rooms.

A sincere thanks to Sandra Daugherty, Liz Wright, Stephen Penta, Lindsay Katt, Dirty Lola, Lauren Saville, and Angel Adeyoha, for providing valuable contributions, insights, and inspiration.

To the many anonymous bar and restaurant patrons, Twitter contributors, and passing acquaintances who offered voluminous opinions both solicited and unsolicited.

To the various pseudonymed folks who trusted me with their hearts and bodies over the past couple decades. I learned something from every one of you, and I'm grateful for every experience I had with you, even the rough ones.

To my father, David, for making sure I was the one kindergartener in Catholic school who knew the words "scrotum" and "vulva." To my mother, Betty, for encouraging me to pursue my dreams, though she was probably gunning for "singer/songwriter." To my sister, Adrienne, and bro-in-law, Ken, for being proud of my sexual activism before I even knew what I was doing.

To Reid Mihalko, for consistently demonstrating unparalleled integrity of character, resilience, and patience. You are my anchor and my lighthouse. This book, like so much good in my life, would simply not exist without you.

ABOUT THE AUTHOR

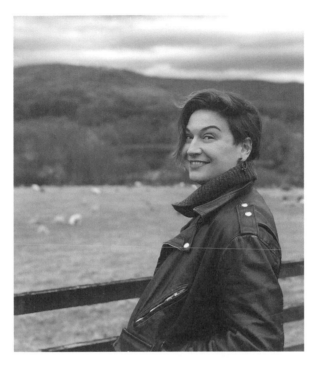

Allison Moon is the author of five books, including the award-winning sex-ed guide *Girl Sex 101*, *Getting It: A Guide to Hot, Healthy Hookups and Shame-Free Sex*, and the erotic memoir *Bad Dyke*. Allison is a popular sex-educator who has presented her workshops—on strap-on sex, cunnilingus, polyamory, sexual self expression, and more—to thousands of people around the United States and Canada. She currently lives with her partner in Oregon at the base of an active volcano.

INDEX

A

abortion, 201, 204–5
abstinence, 251
abuse, 220, 235, 241–42, 257–59
active listening, 119
addictions, 249–50. *See also* alcohol;
    drugs; sex addiction
aftercare, 133–34
alcohol, 139–43, 147
anonymous sex, 162–63
antidepressants, 146
apologies, 153–54
Appreciation Sandwich, 127–28, 129
apps, 169–70
asexuality, 252
attachment styles, 222
attractiveness, 51–54
awkwardness, 61–62

B

baggage, 83
barriers, 193–94
BDSM, 4, 188, 241, 246, 257
birth control, 199–204
blackouts, 139–40
blanket yes, 130
body language, 62
boner pills, 146
booty calls, 163–64
boundaries
    articulating, 19, 107
    in bed, 108–9
    diagram of, 107–8
    drugs and, 145
    holding firm to, 80–81
    meaning of, 107
    violations of, 151–55
breakups, 233–39

C

casual sex
    Bill of Rights, 17
    meaning of, 2–3
    motivations for, 13–15

nonmonogamy and, 226–28
risk assessment and, 187–89
styles of, 159–66
See also sex
celibacy, 251–52
cervical caps, 202
checking in, 103–4, 124–25, 160
chemistry, 60–61, 72
chlamydia, 191, 195
choices
    assessing, 39
    learning from bad, 36–37
    making good, 33–36
clitoris, anatomy of, 180
closet, staying in the, 258
codependence, 221
communication
    Appreciation Sandwich, 127–28, 129
    checking in, 103–4, 124–25, 160
    Difficult Conversation Formula,
        105–6, 152
    dirty talk, 128–29, 174–77
    disclosures, 77–78, 105–7, 195–96
    importance of, 20, 95, 264–65
    language and, 19
    lapses in, 151
    post-coital, 133–36
    requests, 121–22
    sexting, 170–74
    speaking up, 125
    See also consent; "no"; "yes"
community standards, 257–58
compliments, 62
compulsions, 249–50
condoms, 193, 202, 203
consent
    active listening and, 119
    alcohol and, 139–40, 142–43
    chemistry and, 61
    emotional, 101–2
    enthusiastic, 97, 99–101
    informed, 97, 101
    meaning of, 97–98
    silence vs., 66
    See also "no"; "yes"

Library of Congress Cataloging-in-Publication Data
Names: Moon, Allison, author.
Title: Getting it : a guide to hot, healthy hookups and shame-free sex /
Allison Moon.
Description: First edition. | New York : Ten Speed Press, [2020] | Includes
bibliographical references and index.
Identifiers: LCCN 2020021872 (print) | LCCN 2020021873 (ebook) |
ISBN 9781984857156 (trade paperback) | ISBN 9781984857163 (ebook)
Subjects: LCSH: Sex. | Sexual ethics. | Dating (Social customs) |
Communication and sex. | Sexual health.
Classification: LCC HQ31 .M687 2020 (print) | LCC HQ31 (ebook) |
DDC 306.7--dc23
LC record available at https://lccn.loc.gov/2020021872
LC ebook record available at https://lccn.loc.gov/2020021873

Trade Paperback ISBN: 978-1-9848-5715-6
eBook ISBN: 978-1-9848-5716-3

Printed in Malaysia

Design by Annie Marino
Abstract marble art by Bibadash/Shutterstock.com
Speckled terrazzo art by Melissa Wiederrecht/Shutterstock.com

10 9 8 7 6 5 4 3 2

First Edition